Issues in Accident and Emergency Nursing

Issues in Accident and Emergency Nursing

Edited by

Lynn Sbaih

Department of Health Care Studies
Manchester Metropolitan University
Manchester
UK

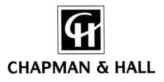

CHAPMAN & HALL

London · Glasgow · Weinheim · New York · Tokyo · Melbourne · Madras

Published by Chapman & Hall, 2–6 Boundary Row, London SE1 8HN, UK

Chapman & Hall, 2–6 Boundary Row, London SE1 8HN, UK

Blackie Academic & Professional, Wester Cleddens Road, Bishopbriggs, Glasgow G64 2NZ, UK

Chapman & Hall GmbH, Pappelallee 3, 69469 Weinheim, Germany

Chapman & Hall Inc., One Penn Plaza, 41st Floor, New York NY 10119, USA

Chapman & Hall Japan, Thomson Publishing Japan, Hirakawacho Nemoto Building, 6F, 1–7–11 Hirakawa-cho, Chiyoda-ku, Tokyo 102, Japan

Chapman & Hall Australia, Thomas Nelson Australia, 102 Dodds Street, South Melbourne, Victoria 3205, Australia

Chapman & Hall India, R. Seshadri, 32 Second Main Road, CIT East, Madras 600 035, India

Distributed in the USA and Canada by Singular Publishing Group Inc., 4284 41st Street, San Diego, California 92105

First edition 1994

© 1994 Chapman & Hall

Typeset in 10/12 Palatino by Mews Photosetting, Beckenham, Kent
Printed in Great Britain by T.J. Press (Padstow) Ltd, Padstow, Cornwall

ISBN 0 412 49830 8   1 56593 184 X (USA)

A catalogue record for this book is available from the British Library

Library of Congress Catalog Card Number: 94-70921

∞ Printed on permanent acid-free text paper, manufactured in accordance with ANSI/NISO Z39.48-1992 and ANSI/NISO Z39.48-1984 (Permanence of Paper).

For Eyad

If a man will begin with certainties he shall end in doubts, but if he will be content to begin with doubts, he will end with certainties.

The Advancement of Learning
Francis Bacon, 1st Baron Verulam (1561–1626)
English writer, philosopher and statesman

Contents

Contributors

Kate Burgess RGN, A and E Manager, Southend Hospital, Essex.

Roberta Burton RGN, ENB 995, Nursing Development Unit Facilitator for the Royal Hospitals, Belfast.

Simon Davies BN (Hons), RGN, DCR, ATNC(P), Trauma Research Fellow, Department of Emergency and Disaster Medicine, Keele University, and Staff Nurse, Emergency Department, North Staffordshire Hospital, Stoke on Trent.

Janet Dutton BA, RGN, ENB 199, Special Projects Officer (Research), North Lincolnshire Health Authority District Headquarters, Lincoln.

Steve Edgeley RMN, DipN, Clinical Nurse Specialist, Liaison Psychiatry, Leicester General Hospital, Leicester.

Lisa Hadfield-Law RGN, A&E Certificate, ATNC (I), TNCC (P), Independent Consultant and Chairperson, ATNC Steering Committee.

Gill Hall RGN, CertEd, RNT, ENB 199, Course Teacher, ENB 199 A&E Nursing, School of Health Studies, Aintree Hospital, Liverpool.

Alison Hopwood RGN, ENB 199, Senior Staff Nurse, Emergency Department, North Staffordshire Hospital, Stoke on Trent.

Chris Jones BA, RGN, ENB 100, RNT, Course Teacher ENB 125, Intensive and Coronary Care Nursing, School of Health Studies, Aintree Hospital, Liverpool.

Paul Kingston RNMH, RMN, MA (Gerontology), CertEd, Research Fellow, Department of Applied Social Studies, University of Keele.

Adele McKenna RGN, ENB 199, Staff Nurse, Emergency Department, North Staffordshire Hospital, Stoke on Trent.

Dave Rowell RMN, EN(M), Clinical Nurse Specialist, Psychiatric Liaison, Leicester General Hospital, Leicester.

Lynn Sbaih BSc(Hons), RGN, RMN, ENB 199, Senior Lecturer, Department of Health Studies, Manchester Metropolitan University, Manchester.

Ian Wood RGN, ENB 199, TNCC(P), ENB 998, Charge Nurse, Emergency Department, North Staffordshire Hospital Centre, Stoke on Trent.

Cherine Woolwich RGN, ONC, A&E Cert, Sister, St Mary's Hospital, Praed Street, London.

Acknowledgements

Thanks are due to all who have contributed to this book and given an ongoing commitment of time and energy.

Thanks are also due to the many who have listened to ideas and provided support and advice during the months of the book's growth.

An introduction and guide to the use of this book

This book is different. It is not a traditional nursing text book but there is something for everyone interested in the development of nursing and delivery of patient care within the A and E department.

The general aims of the book are simple. Issues of current interest to nurses working in A and E have been explored from a number of standpoints. The reader is invited to think about and if necessary challenge the standpoints, ideas and issues put forward and consider all within their own clinical area of practice.

The book has been written for those nurses who are comfortable with the concept of A and E nursing but want to explore some of the issues further. Topics that are addressed are varied and include the ethical debate surrounding triage, the care of children and the elderly in A and E and the introduction of technology. Those with an interest in trauma will also find plenty to keep them happy.

Non A and E nurses, pre- and postregistration nurses visiting A and E to work for short periods of time or those from areas that liaise with the A and E department will find the book useful as a 'dip in' reference book. However, it should be noted that for some chapters where the contributor has made assumptions about the level of knowledge and expertise of the reader, supplementary texts and/or the assistance of experienced A and E nurses may be required as the reader works through the text.

The book is made up of a selection of papers within a number of highly individualized chapters which offer the reader brief but comprehensive reviews of subjects by contributors who view A and E nursing in a number of distinct ways. Readers should therefore expect to find many different views, standpoints and approaches to the presentation of material. Organization of the book's content in this way has resulted in minimal cross-reference between chapters although recurring themes have emerged. Such a format was considered a valuable way of presenting information within the book and purposely sought. It is hoped that exposure to individual chapters within the book will encourage readers to consider issues and problems from perspectives other than the ones with which they are familiar and perhaps comfortable. The reader is then responsible for the consideration, adoption or challenge to the content of any chapter.

During the process of exploration of content, reference should always be made to its potential place within clinical practice and its influence upon the delivery of patient and family care. Although it is acknowledged that each A and E department is different and that the environment and local resources affect the translation of theory into practice, questioning and subsequent challenge of the environment, work issues and ideas should help the reader to widen the debate about nursing in A and E and its anticipated growth into the next century. The intended outcome of such analysis by the reader may be to challenge practice. Alternatively information presented within the book may support or enhance work currently being undertaken within a number of A and E departments.

With reference to the format, the book is not intended to be read from cover to cover. Instead the reader will find the book a valuable source of information that can be dipped into when required, a book where the sampling of arguments put forward by various contributors can be considered. Alternatively the presence of themes within the book makes reading from cover to cover valuable also.

It is acknowledged that some readers may feel that important issues have been omitted. Unfortunately this illustrates that this particular book cannot cover all issues considered to be of importance to all A and E nurses at the current time. To overcome this, the book should be used in conjunction with other books and journals. In addition it is anticipated that the text will be used with other supplementary reading as a stepping stone to the development of more knowledge and ideas which can then be considered in the reader's area of practice. To assist the reader in the development of ideas presented within the book, all contributors supply a reference list at the end of their chapter.

Information within the book may challenge the reader's expectations and more questions than answers may be found, particularly for those seeking specific answers to specific questions. However there is a wealth of information within the book and the contributors, all of whom are familiar with the A and E setting, have discussed issues from what they consider to be a pertinent point of importance.

The outcome of such an approach is the creation of a number of perspectives that present two challenges to the reader. The first challenge is for the reader to consider carefully what each contributor has to say for, as stated earlier, information may be presented from a standpoint different to their own. The second part of the challenge is to translate some of the ideas and standpoints presented within the book into the reader's own area of clinical practice, whether this be a small, medium or large A and E department. The understanding is that all A and E departments accept patients with various injuries and illnesses and for this reason there is something for everyone in this book.

Common themes that have emerged within the book include the concept and use of nursing triage, reflection of the community in A and E, doing and thinking, custom and practice and communication. All chapters attempt to ask questions about individual accountability of the A and E nurse in relation to various debates.

With reference to the theme of 'doing and thinking' in A and E, all contributors have considered the reasons for 'doing' nursing in A and E rather than the 'doing' of A and E nursing only. Often it is easier to measure what is achieved when physical actions and their responses can be observed. However, there are many other actions and reactions that relate to feelings, beliefs, attitudes, past experience and personal judgments. All contributors have been sympathetic to this aspect of A and E nursing.

The theme of custom and practice within A and E also emerges within the book. It is acknowledged that in some departments aspects of care assessment, planning, intervention and evaluation may be determined by custom and practice. Daily work organization, the management of the environment and people may rely upon knowledge of routines associated with doctors, other personnel or the departmental cleaning. Role definition by A and E nurses is part of the challenge to custom, practice and the subsequent time spent in care delivery within the A and E department. All contributors have addressed these issues to some extent within their chapters.

Another issue that emerges from many of the chapters of this book is that of communication and how it underpins the practice of nursing in A and E. Communication is discussed in a number of ways but all references to communication eventually return to the need for A and E nurses to listen to themselves, their colleagues, the nursing press, the patients and their family and friends. Communication with the local community is also addressed by many of the contributors, illustrating a need for nurses to be aware of the society served by the A and E department.

All themes within the book aim to encourage deliberation of the components and scope of the role of the nurse in A and E. It is also acknowledged that a multidisciplinary approach to care assessment, planning, implementation and evaluation is to be strived for within the A and E department.

To assist the reader when dipping into the book, the beginning of each chapter has a brief introduction. The introduction discusses the aim and specific organization of the chapter including a brief description of subject areas covered and explanation relating to how the contributor has tackled issues put forward within the chapter.

When dipping into various chapters, the reader should note that the use of different styles and viewpoints has led to various methods of illustrating arguments. For example, the chapter which explores the use of nursing triage in A and E uses case studies to illustrate points made. This is a very different approach to the chapter on children which revisits much well-known information and illustrates this with drawings from children who have visited one particular A and E department. All approaches used by contributors provide a valuable insight into how information may be presented and all provide a basis for analysis of theory and its associated practice by the reader. Contributors for Chapters 7 and 9 have provided appendices which can be found at the back of the book.

It is acknowledged that what is considered important to the contributor may not be important to the reader and the reader is invited to join the debate through the discussion points available in all chapters. Discussion points are always introduced before the related information is presented. It is then left up to the reader to pursue any questions raised within the discussion points or to leave alone. The goal of discussion points is to present an alternative point of view and raise awareness of certain portions of chapter content. Many discussion points invite the reader to consider and formulate their own questions about practice in relation to the introduced information, the outcome of which should then be development of the debate within the reader's own department.

There is no obligation on the part of the reader to follow the discussion points but there is an obligation to enter the debate just as there is a duty on the part of the contributors within this book to disseminate information and ideas. If neither is done then the growth of A and E nursing may be stunted and this could affect the wishes and needs of practitioners and patients. The reader is therefore urged to consider, in their own area of A and E clinical practice, the ideas to be found within this book.

Formulation of questions and the development of a whole range of debates within A and E departments should help provide challenges to practice. Practice that is being challenged and evaluated can then be supported or eradicated.

In conclusion, professional development of A and E nurses involves the bridging of knowledge acquired through thinking, reflection, discussion, collaboration, reading published literature or attending a course in an educational establishment. Knowledge should be reflected in the delivery of skills. The influence of one upon the other is examined in the chapters of this book.

Information by itself is of limited value unless it can be translated into the practice of nursing in A and E. The contributors expect that everyone reading this book is ready and willing to take ideas into their clinical practice, adapt information and ultimately question clinical practice. The questioning of clinical practice can have two outcomes. Firstly it may be established that what is being practised is sound, safe and acceptable to the patient, family and friends. Alternatively it may be established that some areas of practice require re-evaluation, further discussion and collaboration with other health care colleagues. Whatever the outcome, nurses in A and E will then be in a better position to question their practice, work together as a team and provide a high standard of patient care to all who use the A and E department.

Therefore this book, although different in its organization and intended use, has something for everyone. It is for those who are interested in the development of A and E nurses and nursing. It is for those who wish to evaluate and develop continuity of care to all who use the A and E service. It is for those who wish to consider the relationship of theory and practice in A and E. Whoever the reader may be, issues relating to the delivery and receipt of care in A and E have to be addressed with due regard to the value, skills and knowledge of all involved, including the patient.

A and E nursing is undergoing rapid, explosive change and the right question at the right time in the right place should be viewed as a positive development of current A and E nursing. This book is an acknowledgement of this approach.

CHAPTER 1

The emergency nurse practitioner

A. McKenna, C. Woolwich and K. Burgess

INTRODUCTION

The role of the emergency nurse practitioner is on the verge of changing the face of A and E nursing or plunging into oblivion. This chapter is primarily concerned with the current and developing role of the ENP and information presented is controversial and potentially problematic for the reader. This is due to the chapter being written by three people who view the role of the ENP in three different ways. Tackling the chapter from different perspectives provides a wealth of information as well as approaches to arguments from different standpoints.

The contributors make no apologies for the introduction of many perspectives. They believe that if the role of the ENP is to be developed that it is up to the reader to consider the information presented in relation to their own A and E department. Ultimately this means that it is up to the reader to decide the future of the ENP in A and E; the answer will not be found in this chapter.

The organization of the chapter is such that the scene is set for the reader prior to areas of debate taking place. For example, the role and its potential place in A and E is introduced before a historical stance is taken. Another example is the introduction of the concept of triage as a basis for the debate surrounding the role of the ENP and triage nurse.

An area of recognized controversy within the chapter is that of training and the debate focuses upon the local versus national training needs and the concerns of those involved in preparation of ENPs for A and E related practice. As with all chapters in this book the reader is not expected to agree with information and arguments put forward. Information is to be considered via questions raised in the discussion points. In addition it is expected that other information in the chapter will be challenged by the reader as necessary.

The reader may also feel that important points have been omitted. For example, the contributors have used the American model of the ENP upon which to base their ideas and suggest ways of development for the British ENP. There is little mention of models from other countries.

Finally, information within the chapter has been organized in sections which are designed to be dipped into or read in relation to other sections. The reader should find the chapter useful as a reference chapter as well as one that can be read from start to finish.

DEFINING THE ROLE

There is a clear need for an agreed definition of the role of the emergency nurse practitioner (ENP). To this end the Emergency Nurse Practitioner Special Interest Group (RCN, 1992), under the auspices of the Accident and Emergency Nurses Association, has defined the role in the following way:

An emergency nurse practitioner (ENP) is an Accident and Emergency nurse who has a sound nursing practice base in all aspects of Accident and Emergency nursing, with formal post-basic education in holistic assessment, in physical diagnosis, in prescription of treatment and in the promotion of health.

The emergency nurse practitioner is:

- a key member of the emergency health care team
- directly available to members of the public
- an autonomous practitioner, able to assess, diagnose, treat and discharge patients without reference to a doctor but within prearranged guidelines.

The concept of a nurse practising in an autonomous role is not new to the profession in the United Kingdom. Nurses in other areas such as in the community have for many years had the status and legal responsibility of an autonomous practitioner (Stilwell, 1982). More recently this concept has been extended into the Accident and Emergency department and an autonomous practitioner role has been developing for some years. The role was pioneered at Oldchurch Hospital, Essex in 1983 (Ramsden, 1986).

The ENP is seen as an autonomous practitioner. This term implies that the ENP should be able to consult with and prescribe care for patients without automatic referral to a doctor. The ENP should also be able to refer the patient to other agencies, such as the A and E doctor, dentist, general practitioner, community nurse, chiropodist or drug addiction agency as the need arises.

It has been stated that all nurses practising in the sphere of A and E could be regarded as ENPs (Walsh, 1989). The same author suggests that to function as an autonomous practitioner the A and E nurse would have to be able to justify all actions with sound reason and research findings and implies that this would be a daunting task. The RCN Special Interest Group has indicated that the role holder should have a sound nursing practice base, which is defined as the experience gained by 'a minimum of three years of continuous clinical exposure to A and E nursing and the acknowledgement of that exposure by other A and E colleagues'.

Education

There are two schools of thought. Oldchurch Hospital (Ramsden, 1986) suggested that the role of the ENP could be undertaken by a registered nurse with five years or more experience and no formal postregistration education required. However, others recommend that a formal period of postregistration training is essential in order to practise as an ENP (see also Training required on page 22).

Points for discussion

- Should the emergency nurse practitioner be autonomous?
- Can all nurses practising in the sphere of A and E be regarded as emergency nurse practitioners?
- Is experience required for the role?
- Is formal postregistration education necessary for the role?

A NEED FOR THE ROLE?

In some inner city areas in the UK, the demand for primary health care in the community is greater than the services available. The resulting vacuum is being filled by the local A and E departments. In addition, there are problems of both medical and nursing staffing within these departments (James and Pyrgos, 1989).

As demands upon the service have grown and changed, so those supplying the service have had to contemplate changes to their traditional working practice. Nursing has much to offer the currently stressed health care system (Fagin, 1982). One avenue that has been tested is the introduction of ENPs.

The large numbers of patients who attend A and E when in fact hospital attendance is not a clinical necessity have prompted strenuous attempts to devise solutions to this problem. Amongst these suggestions has been the mooted introduction of GPs resident in A and E departments (James and Pyrgos, 1989). However, this might serve to exacerbate rather than alleviate the problem: if patients know that by going to A and E they are guaranteed a prompt consultation with a GP, they may not be encouraged to seek help more appropriately elsewhere.

In the long term, an alternative would be to boost the available community services to the point where patients' expectations can be met through these services rather than by attending A and E. Examples of this are the Leek Moorlands Memorial Hospital in Staffordshire and the Ramsey Cottage Hospital on the Isle of Man.

The policy of nurse-run community treatment centres is also being taken up by health authorities whose smaller A and E departments, often in inner city areas, are under threat of closure. This is as a response to the centralization of health care resources at local levels (Simon, 1992). Certain patients can be offered a choice between consulting either a doctor or a nurse. It has been suggested that this choice allows a more patient centred approach to care and the overall quality of the service provided to the patient may be improved as a direct result (Andrews, 1988).

Although difficult, measuring quality of care is very important so that health professionals' performance may be compared to expectation. American research of ENP effectiveness is extensive and studies indicate that in their clinical capabilities, productivity and quality of care, nurse practitioners are comparable to first year medical staff (Sox, 1979; Salkever et al., 1982). In some studies patients being cared for by ENPs alone progressed better than those under doctors' care (Lewis and Resnick, 1967; Spitzer et al., 1974).

In the interim, however, the ENP can contribute invaluably to the management of this group of patients. Not only are they in a position to prescribe and carry out the minor treatments required but by dint of their nursing training and unique frontline position in patient care, they are possibly ideally placed to advise, educate and refer these patients to more appropriate sources of care if necessary. Yet another alternative that could be considered is the provision of community treatment room facilities staffed by ENPs (Simon, 1992). The hours of service could be offered to meet local needs. Referrals to the A and E departments or to GPs might be arranged by ENPs if appropriate. Such a service may relieve some of the pressures in local A and E departments whilst those patients who choose to be seen in a community treatment room could also be seen, arguably more appropriately, away from the A and E environment. This is not a new idea. Beloff and Paris in 1967 suggested that overuse of A and E departments reflected the 'malfunctioning of the community health care system' and said that a solution to the problem would have to be found 'outside the hospital'. ENPs, either working as educators within the A and E department or in community treatment centres, may be a possible interim solution until more widespread upgrading of community health care provision becomes feasible.

It is already the case that in some community hospitals, nursing staff provide an emergency service for minor injuries in areas where the nearest district A and E department is some considerable distance away. Better use can be made of nurse time because for some patients the ENP is able to prescribe treatment which can be carried out by herself or other nurses, without the need for a doctor to intervene (Jones, 1986). It has also been demonstrated that there is an increase in job satisfaction for the role holder who is able to make independent decisions for patient care (Rice, 1989; Burgess, 1992).

At present there are undoubtedly a significant proportion of patients attending A and E departments nationwide who could perfectly safely be seen and treated by a suitably qualified nurse. By treating these patients using ENPs, they are effectively removed from the number of those who have to wait to see the A and E doctor. The ENP is able to fulfil a function in releasing medical staff to deal with patients who are more seriously ill and injured and in most need of prompt medical attention (Woolwich, 1992). The domino effect of this means that seriously ill patients are receiving the best possible care, whilst the ENP, by autonomously diagnosing, treating and discharging those attending with minor injuries, is offering them an ideal treatment path if they so wish.

Waiting times

Possibly the primary impetus for the establishment of ENPs in A and E departments in the UK has been the steadily increasing attendances at such departments (Jones, 1986; James and Pyrgos, 1989). These lead in turn to increased patient waiting times across all triage groups and most particularly for patients attending with minor injuries.

It has been suggested that some of these patients could be offered the choice of consulting an experienced and appropriately trained nurse who could safely 'fast track' them through the system, avoiding excessive waiting times (Woolwich, 1992). Numerous authors claim to have demonstrated that provision of an ENP service does have significant benefits in terms of waiting time reductions (James and Pygros, 1989; Burgess, 1992; Head, 1988). Unsurprisingly in view of this body of evidence, many departments are examining the concept of or are in the process of establishing an ENP service.

Whilst hard to quantify, there is anecdotal evidence of an increase in waiting room hostility aimed primarily towards staff in the A and E department (Rice, 1989). This is possibly an inevitable consequence of the overburdening of A and E facilities and lengthening waiting times. The presence of a suitably qualified staff member able to give advice and reassurance as well as carry out agreed treatments and arrange investigations might serve to alleviate this phenomenon.

The result of consumer surveys carried out in A and E departments over a wide area of the UK led to the conclusion that many patients have unrealistic expectations of the A and E service (Fawcett-Henesy, 1990). Many patients expect to be seen rapidly for a huge variety of minor injuries (Lewis and Bradbury, 1982) often knowing that they require merely a simple dressing or tetanus immunization booster. Often these patients can become quite upset on learning that a lengthy wait to see a doctor may be required of them, which they may feel to be unnecessary. It may be that the establishment of an ENP service staffed by A and E nurses able to deal with such problems would meet the expectations of this group of patients. Patients also attend the A and E department simply to seek advice from someone with recognized knowledge and experience. Again the ENP could be viewed as such a person and might be able to meet this requirement. Interestingly, there is a high degree of patient satisfaction with existing ENP schemes and the vast majority of patients who have experienced the service are happy to be assessed and treated by an ENP (Head, 1988).

The ENP is in a good position to act as an instructor in health care and prevention of injury and illness. Patients who attend the A and E department with conditions or injuries suitable for treatment by the ENP will come into contact with a health care professional whose background is very different from that of a doctor. Nurses already give practical care, advice and provide some degree of health education in a model of self-care (Tettersall, 1988). It has been suggested that nurses have better communication skills than doctors and are able to lend a listening ear (Walsh, 1989). The same author believes that the establishment of an ENP role might allow the A and E nurse to further develop skills in counselling, health education and preventive medicine.

The ENP post may offer A and E nurses the opportunity to fulfil a much more defined health education function covering accident prevention, advice on first aid and information about the correct use of GP and community services (Aiken, 1982). A and E nurses might also become involved in initiatives to provide health care to the homeless and in the provision of specific health education in relation to drug and alcohol dependency. It should be noted, however, that the skills of the ENP should be complementary to those of their medical colleagues, rather than interchangeable with them. It has been found that nurses are often regarded as more approachable than doctors and are also more inclined to look at a patient's psychosocial needs as well as their physical problems. Indeed, there is evidence that some groups of people such as the elderly, women and certain minority groups, especially Asian women, will consult more readily with a nurse than with a doctor (Tettersall, 1988).

The establishment of an ENP post therefore ought to make these special abilities of A and E nurses more immediately accessible to the patient. Ten years ago it was suggested that in some clinical contexts it might be appropriate to expand the nurse's role to ensure an adequate distribution of services (Pearson, 1983). It would seem that the evolution of the ENP role in A and E has been a major move in that direction.

Points for discussion

- Does the ENP role provide patient focused care and patient choice, thereby improving the quality of service?

- Can the ENP redirect patients to a more appropriate source of care if necessary?

- Will the ENP enable better use of available nursing and medical resources?

- Is there a need to find a way of reducing waiting times across all triage groups?

- Can the ENP help to reduce waiting room hostility?

- Can the ENP close the gap between patient expectations and actual experience?

- Will the introduction of ENPs enhance opportunities for health education and accident prevention?

HISTORY AND DEVELOPMENT OF THE ROLE

The role of the ENP is still evolving and ever more opportunities are opening for A and E nurses (Gould, 1988). In this section the origins of the service will be outlined and the impetus behind the establishment of the role will be examined.

Independent autonomous nurse specialists outside the UK are not a new development. They have been a fact of life in the USA since the early 1970s (Aiken, 1982). In the aftermath of the Vietnam war, many medical corpsmen were returning to positions as physician's assistants, working in areas undersupplied with medical resources (Bowling, 1987). The nursing profession, seeing the work of a physician's assistant as encroaching upon their traditional roles, developed their own specialist role, that of the nurse practitioner (NP).

Initially the role of the NP was pioneered to provide adequate ambulatory care to patients in rural areas and to augment the primary health care services provided by medical practitioners in such areas (Geolot, Alongis and Edlich, 1977). ENPs began to appear for several reasons: doctors became more interested in specialist career paths rather than general medical practice; the inaccessibility of medical care at night and on weekends; and the mobile nature of the population (Geolot, 1987). As a consequence there was an increase in attendances at emergency rooms and those practitioners still working in rural areas experienced an increased burden of visits.

In the UK, nurses working in an independent and semiautonomous role have long been present in the form of community midwives, district nurses and health visitors. Many of these specialist community nurses have explored ways of improving services and, in particular, making them more responsive to patients' needs (Salvage, 1990). As a corollary to this the development of an autonomous nurse practitioner role in general practice is now well established (Stilwell, 1982).

From an A and E perspective, nurses working in small minor casualties across the country have been practising unrecognized as independent practitioners for many years (Stilwell, 1982). A study in Wessex as long ago as 1974 showed that whilst less than 1% of patients attending A and E in district hospitals were seen by a nurse alone, in peripheral hospitals staffed by nurses and GPs, over 60% were treated by a nurse alone (Cliff, 1974). Many such nurse and GP-run clinics still offer ambulatory services today and the staff who work in them can reasonably be regarded as the true pioneers of the emergency nurse practitioner role in the UK.

ENPs: the UK experience

Nurses were first formally accorded the title of emergency nurse practitioner in a trial organized by Oldchurch Hospital in Essex (Ramsden, 1986). Though the job they were performing could be regarded as an evolution of that performed by many of the sisters and nurses previously alluded to working in small departments, there were major differences. The establishment of the role in this case was at the instigation of the Community Health Council and was subject to a number of strict guidelines, relating to criteria of patients whom the ENP could treat and also investigations that they could order (Head, 1988). Since that original UK experience, further pioneering work has been done in Southend Hospital in Essex, Derby Royal Infirmary, Lincoln County Hospital, St Mary's Hospital in London and others. Today the role is developing apace.

Points for discussion

● Is the ENP a cheap alternative to a doctor?

● Could the ENP become a doctor substitute?

● Is the ENP a uniquely nursing role?

It has been suggested that amongst the reasons for establishing an ENP service is that ENPs can do a doctor's tasks more cheaply (Warden, 1988). There are a number of ways in which such misconceptions of the role may have arisen. In part, because of the difficulties inherent in establishing such a new role as the ENP, there has been a trend to try and define the responsibilities of an ENP in terms of discrete tasks that may be performed. This, indeed, seems to be a problem not just confined to the ENP role: Lewis and Bradbury (1982) described a study which showed that A and E nurses generally were unable to identify their role in the emergency department, tending to perceive it in terms of medically designated functions (Tooley and Field, 1985). ENPs should be aware that using medical models of illness and a task orientated approach may eventually lead to restrictive and narrow parameters of practice.

Historically, ENPs have to some extent been regarded as doctor substitutes (James and Pygros, 1989). Whilst this is not a view supported by the RCN (1992), nonetheless the temptation still exists to use ENPs to address specific tasks and organize prescribed and agreed investigations to aid the doctor in a medical work-up. In America it has even been advocated that nurse practitioners be employed in hospital posts as direct replacements for resident junior doctors (Silver and McAtee, 1988).

It falls to ENPs themselves and the nursing profession generally to stress the unique nursing qualities of the role and to avoid strict adherence to fixed illness and task orientated medical approaches. If such approaches continue to be followed, it may very well be that the medical profession will control the evolution of what is essentially a new development in nursing. If nurses working as ENPs find themselves regarded merely as A and E doctors' assistants, satisfaction with the role may be adversely affected.

PARAMETERS OF PRACTICE

The precise role and responsibilities of A and E nurses employed as ENPs will be defined by the parameters of practice within which they work.

There are currently no nationally agreed parameters of practice. As a result, individual A and E departments have set up posts tailored to meet their individual needs, according to patient attendance profiles and staff capabilities. It is, however, possible to give a general outline of the role and parameters to which ENPs may work. Table 1.1 covers the parameters of practice a typical ENP may be working to. These are very similar across the country.

Table 1.1: A typical example of parameters of practice for ENPs

- Minor injuries to the extremeties (including grazes, lacerations, burns and scalds)
- Minor eye injuries/complaints
- Patients requiring tetanus immunization only
- Removal of foreign bodies (including those from ears and noses)
- Treatment of uncomplicated stings and insect bites
- Treatment of minor head injuries
- Patients requiring reassurance and or advice on a medical problem
- Prescription of investigations, e.g. X-ray

It should be noted that the precise guidelines for ENPs will vary; not all ENPs will be expected to cover all these groups of patients and there may be other tasks performed by some ENPs which are not detailed in Table 1.1. The table serves only as an amalgam of practice from a variety of departments and should not be taken to precisely represent the policies to which any given ENP works.

Initially when an ENP role is being established, the competence of individuals working in the ENP role must be fully assessed. This can be facilitated by having, initially, very restrictive parameters for practice. As the role holder gains experience and can be shown by internal audit to practise safely, it may well be possible to permit expansion of the scope of ENP practice within a given A and E department.

As there are no nationally agreed parameters for ENP practice, individual A and E units have to devise them for themselves, as mentioned earlier. Usually guidelines to which an ENP works will be arrived at by a consultative process, as a result of agreement between a variety of interested and affected parties. Indeed, acceptance by all health care workers with whom the ENP interacts is crucial for the ENP role implementation (Widhalm and Anderson, 1982). These may include other A and E nursing and medical colleagues affected by the practice of the ENP, such as the orthopaedic and radiology departments. Hospital management and the nursing practice advisory committee should also be included.

Review of the parameters of practice

It would be facile and arrogant of the authors to suggest a timetable for this process. Individual A and E units are probably those best placed to decide when there is a need for review. There may be changes in staff numbers or make-up which necessitate expansion or reduction in the number of patient categories which the ENP should be seeing. Similarly, the proportions of patients attending with different injuries may vary with time: an area once a major industrial producer or mining town with many industrial accidents may experience an all too rapid progression to a region where few are employed and such accidents become less common. Therefore to best utilize the practitioner's abilities, in such an area it might be necessary to increase the scope of the ENP's role. Consequently the parameters of practice are probably best reviewed, extended or otherwise changed as and when necessary to meet the changing needs of the community or the A and E department.

A hint of this has been given in the discussion put forward for why the parameters should be subject to review. Individual A and E units may be serving widely different communities or have different staffing levels. For example, one hospital may regularly receive many patients with eye injuries and it is appropriate for ENPs working in that department to be sufficiently trained to be able to deal with these patients. Alternatively, a second A and E unit may be located in a city with a specialist eye casualty unit and so see very few patients with eye injuries as an isolated presentation. In this instance, further training in management of eye injuries for the ENPs might not be deemed appropriate.

Thus, by looking at the patient profile of A and E units and the existing talents of staff working as ENPs in these units, the general parameters outlined in Table 1.1 can be specifically formed to meet the needs of the communities concerned.

Points for discussion

● How restrictive should parameters of practice be?

● How are parameters of practice decided?

● How often should parameters of practice be reviewed?

● How can parameters of practice be adapted for departments?

DUTIES AND RESPONSIBILITIES

These may be divided into clinical, managerial and professional areas and should allow for the full potential of the role to develop.

The primary clinical responsibilities of the ENP must include the assessment of the nature and extent of selected patients' injuries/complaints, the establishing of a diagnosis and the prescription of the necessary treatment.

In order to carry these out effectively the authority to order and the knowledge to evaluate agreed diagnostic studies must be included as part of the ENP's duties. The parameters of practice may require the ENP to perform and monitor some therapeutic procedures and these should be clearly stated. Arranging the subsequent management and follow-up of such cases is also the responsibility of the ENP.

There needs to be agreement with medical staff regarding the administration of prescribed medication. Current practice makes use of protocols or standing orders using an approved drug list.

Managerial responsibilities should include the maintenance of detailed and accurate patient records, the effective management of the workload and any other related commitments. There may be a responsibility for the maintenance and collation of statistics pertaining to the post in order to assess its effectiveness and aid in audit or research.

Professional components might include referral to the medical staff of any patient whose complaint/injury is found to fall outside the agreed parameters of practice and the promotion and maintenance of good professional relationships within the department, hospital and community. The ENP assumes accountability for all actions whilst undertaking the responsibilities of the ENP. The nurse is also responsible for personal and professional development and should attend in-service training and/or external courses relevant to areas of expertise.

This outline is incomplete and as such should not be seen as a comprehensive list for those wishing to include such a section within an ENP job description. However, it serves as an indication of what is involved in the role. It acknowledges the scope of practice and autonomy of the role, as well as the responsibility and accountability of the nurse (Becker *et al.*, 1989).

Some of the duties are self-explanatory and need little elaboration; for instance, the need to maintain accurate patient records and documentation. It is accepted that detailed accurate records allow for good communication between staff involved in patient care as well as providing for accurate audit records to be compiled. However, other areas may be considered more contentious and will be dealt with in more detail in the following sections.

In order for the ENP to treat patients adequately, it would seem only reasonable that the ENP be sufficiently well trained to competently assess all those patients whose injuries or illnesses place them within the parameters for ENP practice. However, before a full indepth assessment of patients can be made, it may well be necessary for the patient to undergo a more rapid and superficial screening process such as formal nurse triage.

Triage is the process of sorting patients into priority order for care (Blythin, 1988a, b). It was introduced during World War One as a means of dividing casualties into three categories – those requiring immediate care to save life, those who could wait for care and those beyond help. In 1960 the system was extended to the civilian population of America (Beachley and Snow, 1988). While still used by the military in times of conflict, more recently the process has been adapted by nurses for use in A and E departments worldwide (Jones, 1988).

Triage is the rapid assessment of the patient presenting to the A and E department in order to assess the nature of their complaint or injury, allowing a priority of care to be given based on that assessment (Mallett and Woolwich, 1990). The process should ensure that patients are seen and treated within an appropriate time in an appropriate area of the A and E department. It is an additional nursing skill which relies on the professional judgement of the nurse, for which the nurse is accountable and responsible, as well as adherence to agreed departmental criteria.

Professional nurse triage is always carried out by nursing staff, as opposed to non-professional triage, where a limited sorting process is practised by others: for example clerical admissions staff in waiting areas, ambulance officers or other emergency service workers at a site distant to the A and E department such as in case of major emergencies.

It should be noted that the assessment of a patient carried out by the ENP is not the same as that by a triage nurse. The triage nurse places patients into categories according to the required urgency of treatment. The ENP is required to determine a diagnosis and the precise nature of the required treatment. This process may involve arranging further tests and investigations such as blood tests or X-rays. These two roles are clearly different.

Point for discussion

● Should the ENP be the first nurse to assess patients?

Should the ENP perform triage?

There is some confusion, even within the ranks of A and E nursing, betweeen the roles of nurse triage in A and E and that of the emergency nurse practitioner. As discussed, there appears to be a fundamental difference in the process of assessment carried out by the A and E triage nurse and that of the examination carried out by the ENP.

Patients should be asssessed first by a suitably trained triage nurse and then allocated to see either the A and E doctor or the ENP, with some means to indicate the urgency with which the patient should be seen.

Indeed, some ENPs do not consider it safe practice for one nurse to carry out both the function of an ENP and that of triage concurrently. It is felt that the wearing of two clinical hats may lead to confusion of priorities of care for patients waiting to be triaged (Potter, 1990). On the other hand, many A and E departments are currently facing considerable financial constraints and staffing problems. Understandably this has led some to advocate that the roles of nurse triage and the ENP could and indeed should be combined (Burgess, 1992).

The case for the ENP performing triage

As well as the obvious saving in manpower if only one senior experienced nurse is required to assess and treat patients rather than two, there is another argument in favour of the combined role. The ENP is able to decide at the first assessment of a patient whether their injuries or conditions are suitable for her to treat. If another A and E nurse were to see the patient first and then direct them to see either the A and E doctor or the ENP on duty, two negative results might follow. Firstly, the triaging nurse may send patients to see the ENP whose condition fell outside the ENP's parameters or competence to treat. The ENP would then have to refer the patient on to a doctor. In consequence the patient might become frustrated at being seen by two different nurses, both powerless to resolve the patient's problem. Secondly, the triage nurse might send to the doctor patients who could and should have been treated by an ENP. This may result in unnecessarily lengthy delays for the patient.

The case against the ENP performing triage

In busy A and E departments, the workloads of the ENP and triage nurse can be considerable. There might be the danger that as pressure of work built up, the clinical judgement of the nurse carrying out the role of nurse triage and also working as the ENP might become compromised or confused to the detriment of the patients under their care.

Under the recently introduced Patients Charter (Department of Health, 1991) there is an obligation upon the A and E department for all patients to be seen by a qualified nurse immediately. This could be interpreted as meaning that a superficial assessment should be carried out quickly and carefully by an experienced nurse. This is obviously difficult if the ENP is also performing triage. The role of the ENP is to perform a more thorough examination involving assessment of injuries, requesting investigations if necessary, establishing a diagnosis and prescribing treatments. This leads to concern for the patients who continue to arrive in the department and await triage. They may have to wait a great deal longer than would otherwise be the case if they were triaged by a different nurse first. If a patient arrives with only minor injuries and suffers a long delay in being triaged, whilst contrary to the spirit of the Patients Charter, their treatment is not unduly affected by the delay in initial assessment. If, however, a patient arrives who needs prompt medical attention and the ENP is already involved in a prolonged assessment or treatment of another patient, then the delay in being triaged may put them at an increased risk.

If the A and E nurse is carrying out both roles and is aware that other patients are waiting to be triaged while she is practising in the ENP role, then she may be faced with a dilemma. There might be a temptation to rush the patient currently being treated in order to avoid delay in triaging the waiting patients.

Points for discussion

● What investigations should the ENP be able to arrange?

● What is the position of ENPs in relation to prescribing?

As already discussed, the ENP is empowered to diagnose, treat and discharge patients suffering a variety of injuries and conditions without reference to a doctor. To do this the ENP may well be required to arrange investigations to aid in diagnosis. This autonomy is crucial to the role and also raises very interesting ethical dilemmas, particularly with regard to requesting X-ray investigations and prescribing of medications.

Until recently, radiographers were legally prohibited from accepting requests for X-ray investigation from anyone other than a qualified medical, dental or veterinary practitioner. However, under the revised Radiographers Board Statement of Conduct (CPSM, 1989), with provisos, requesting of limited X-rays by nurses is now legitimate, allowing ENPs to include this task amongst their parameters of practice.

Whilst some see requesting X-rays and interpretation of X-rays as an integral part of the ENP role (Woolwich, 1992), it is as controversial amongst the nursing profession as amongst their medical and radiological colleagues. Other parties feel that it is inappropriate for nurses, even ENPs, to take on such responsibility. Indeed, the issue of X-ray requesting has been a major factor in establishing the unique nature of the ENP role.

Prior to the introduction of ENPs in A and E departments, A and E nurses were not allowed to officially request X-rays and considerable concern was shown by radiology and medical staff in many hospitals when the scheme was introduced (Ramsden, 1986). As a result, such parties have until now had to be convinced by individually run departmental trials and audit of the safety and efficacy of nurses prescribing X-ray investigations. However, there is now a growing body of evidence to show that A and E nurses can and do prescribe safely and comparably with their medical colleagues in A and E (James and Pyrgos, 1989; Woolwich, 1992). Proponents for ENPs requesting and interpreting their own X-ray examinations argue that, as the practitioner examining the patient and completing the request form for X-ray, the ENP is accountable. Part of the X-ray request form requires a provisional diagnosis to be made based on the clinical findings.

Point for discussion

● Is it not then reasonable to allow the ENP to recognize the abnormality, or lack of it, that she or he has thought to confirm by radiological examination?

If ENPs are unable to interpret their own X-rays, requested by themselves, then it may not be appropriate for them to be requesting them in the first place. There is, however, the contrary argument that time savings can be shown, with no detrimental effect on patient care, by nurses prescribing X-rays straight from triage even when these films are reviewed by doctors attending the patient at a later stage (James and Pyrgos, 1989; Rice, 1989; Ramsden, 1986).

However, it would seem crucial to the autonomous role of the ENP that they should be able to act upon the findings of X-rays they have requested. Therefore it seems logical that they should either be adequately trained to interpret the X-rays themselves or that there should be a facility for immediate reporting. The latter would enable the ENP to act upon her diagnosis without reference to an A and E doctor and without detriment to the patient.

Similar arguments can be applied to the need for ENPs to have access to other investigations.

Points for discussion

● Should ENPs be ordering and interpreting blood tests such as full blood counts or urea and electrolytes?

● Should ENPs be sending specimens of urine for microscopy or pregnancy tests?

Fortunately, simply taking a small sample of these fluids is unlikely to be as potentially hazardous as dosing a patient with radiation inherent in radiological examination and therefore there may not be as much resistance to the concept. As is the case for X-rays, the ENP should be adequately trained to interpret and therefore act upon results of tests which they are allowed to organize or else have an immediate interpretation facility available.

It has been advocated that one of the great benefits of an ENP service is that they should be able to prescribe and administer simple analgesia, immunizations, dressings and treatments without the patient having to be seen by a doctor. This poses a considerable ethical problem with prescription of medications and immunizations.

Whilst it has been a matter of debate for some time, there is as yet no legal basis whereby nurses can directly prescribe medications and immunizations on their own cognizance, although situations do exist in some A and E departments whereby written prescription for wound dressings is not required. The BMA and RCN have been discussing nurse prescribing for some time in the wake of the Cumberlege report and others (Cumberlege, 1986).

A and E nurses may already be making decisions on dressing types to be used without written instruction other than 'dressing' written in the A and E notes by attending doctors. When doing this the nurse is exercising judgement on the basis of training and experience. The nurse with limited prescribing rights could be an asset to both the doctor and the patient, as long as these rights are not abused and 'as long as proven, research based care is implemented' (Milward, 1990). Safe prescribing of medications by ENPs would require either very precise guidelines to be rigorously adhered to or sufficient training and awareness of current research and knowledge of pharmacology to allow safe therapeutic prescribing with sound scientific basis. That this is in fact possible is demonstrated by American studies (La Plant and O'Bannol, 1987).

A 'nurse prescribing' bill, primarily for use in the community, is currently going through Parliament, but until the legal situation in the UK with regard to nurse prescribing of medications such as analgesia and oral antibiotics is resolved, avenues are being explored in an endeavour to bypass the restrictions imposed.

Point for discussion

● These legal difficulties can be resolved by use of protocols or 'standing orders' whereby a named ENP is covered to administer or dispense medication that has been prescribed by a doctor as part of the protocol. The protocol sets out the circumstances under which the ENP *must* administer the prescribed dose (Woolwich, 1992). Is this safe, legal and ethical?

Primarily the ENP, as any other nurse, assumes responsibility for his or her own activities. Under the recently introduced *Scope of Professional Practice* (UKCC, 1992) a nurse can accept responsibility for those activities she feels competent and confident to perform. In view of the nature of the ENP role, however, and the fact that ENPs are working within guidelines or parameters defined by the health authority under whose auspices they are employed, there is an additional factor in play. ENPs will normally be covered by their employing authority who will take on vicarious liability for ENPs performing tasks designated to them.

Scope of professional practice and the ENP

For ENPs this new legislation means that once the ENP's practice has been shown to be safe by means of internal audit, roles may be taken on without the need for complicated protocols as described earlier.

Points for discussion

- With what success have nurses working as ENPs established this right for themselves in areas which traditionally have been the province of their medical colleagues?

- Does the *Scope of Professional Practice* (UKCC, 1992) legislation affect the role of the ENP?

The *Scope of Professional Practice* (UKCC, 1992) has been in force for a short period only. As a result, the long term implications cannot be assessed by studying changes wrought in the role so far but will have to be surmised. Theoretically, the new *Scope of Professional Practice* should allow nurses to take greater responsibility for their actions. Provided an adequate training programme can be instigated to enable ENPs to broaden their skills, the legislation should allow expansion of the role to meet needs as and when they become identified. It ought perhaps to be borne in mind, however, that ENPs are nurse practitioners and as such should beware of the dangers of taking over medical tasks purely to relieve pressures on the medical side of A and E staffing.

EMERGENCY NURSE PRACTITIONERS IN THE A AND E DEPARTMENT

Clearly ENPs in A and E are in a unique position. The role has enabled nurses to gain the knowledge, experience and skills to function more effectively (Markham, 1988). Their role is very different to that of other nurses working in A and E. They are able to work as independent practitioners and make autonomous decisions in relation to determining diagnosis and prescribing the appropriate care and treatment. In this context it could be seen as an entirely separate clinical role for A and E nurses utilizing skills beyond those usually thought of as being in the nursing sphere. In representing such a radical change in the traditional role of the nurse, which may in effect be said to redefine nursing practice, it can be regarded as a specialist role. It has been suggested that the clinical nurse specialist should possess leadership abilities and communication skills to function successfully as a nurse consultant (Walker, 1986).

Combining the role of the ENP with the A and E sister

Arguments supporting combination

Some practitioners firmly advocate that the role of the ENP can be carried out as an additional facet of the A and E sister's role. It has been suggested that the A and E sister should be regarded as the true nurse specialist in A and E and master all aspects of A and E nursing. Additionally it has been suggested that fragmentation of the profession by establishing a separate emergency nurse practitioner entity could lead to problems. With stringent financial planning required under the 'opting out' of some NHS hospitals and the establishment of hospital trusts, provision of a 24-hour ENP service using additional staff would prove prohibitively expensive.

The alternative is that all A and E sisters be trained to carry out the duties and fulfil the function of the ENP as part of their total work commitment, that the role of the ENP should therefore be regarded as an integral part of the A and E sister role and that A and E sisters/charge nurses should perform as ENPs when needs demand. Also suggested is that this development would enable the provision of 24-hour, seven days a week ENP cover without the need to hire staff over and above the complement of sisters/charge nurses already present (Burgess, 1992). It should also ensure that there is total commitment and understanding from all sisters for the role. The advocates for combined roles suggest that as a result of this the A and E sister would become the true clinical expert in the A and E department and as such the most valuable manpower asset in A and E nursing.

There are potent arguments to be weighed on both sides of this issue. Those who oppose the combination of the role of the ENP with that of the A and E sister regard the specialist nature of the ENP role to be of utmost importance.

Arguments against combination

These can be summarized by emphasizing a few salient points. As already alluded to, the ENP role represents a radical departure from traditionally accepted A and E nursing practice. It is a role requiring the post holder to shoulder considerable new responsibilities and exercise a wide variety of new skills. As such, some practitioners believe the role of ENP should not be undertaken by junior or even middle grade nursing staff who have still to learn the other skills required of the A and E nurse.

While the provision of a 24-hour ENP service is given as an argument for a combining of roles and may be necessary for some A and E departments, this would not be the case for all. Workloads during the night would need to justify the requirement by each individual department.

The proponents of this argument view the ENP role as a potential career development for experienced nurses wishing to stay in the clinical area, developing and practising new skills. As such it may open up a new career path for nurses whose only opportunity for advancement previously would have been to move into managerial or administrative posts, losing direct patient contact. This pathway of development would lead to the establishment of an ENP role as an additional career tier separate from those in the traditional A and E structure (Woolwich, 1992).

It has also been suggested that a nurse working solely as an ENP would soon lose skills in the latest management of major injuries, resuscitation and A and E procedures, for example, whilst by the same token, A and E sisters would lose their expertise in the field of minor injuries as these groups of patients would all be seen and treated by the ENP. In a sense, then, both A and E sister and the ENP could be regarded as becoming deskilled to some extent but hyperskilled in other areas. Whilst this may occur in departments where ENPs, either through circumstances or choice, carry out other nursing duties in addition to the ENP role, it cannot be employed as an argument against establishing a separate career post of ENP. Such nurses would, after all, only need the skills specific to the ENP role as the A and E sisters would retain responsibility for those whose illness or injuries fell outside the parameters of the ENP's practice.

It may also be argued that dedicated, fulltime ENPs would allow for the role to develop and expand into a more comprehensive service, perhaps not possible if all A and E sisters were to become part-time ENPs.

Points for discussion

● Is the ENP a clinical nurse specialist?

● Can the ENP role be combined with the role of the A and E sister or staff nurse?

● Is deskilling an important issue to be considered for the ENP or A and E sister/staff nurse when taking on the new role?

HOLISTIC CARE AND THE ENP

The term *holistic* is derived from the Greek meaning 'embracing the whole' and in nursing terminology, is taken to imply dealing with all the patient's needs whether they be physical, psychological or social. The special abilities of nurses which so admirably suit them to embracing the concept of holistic care have been discussed earlier.

As the workload of ENPs increases, another dilemma may arise. The ENP may become too busy to carry out all the nursing care, intervention and treatments of all patients they consult with. This might lead to the need for them to delegate some of their workload to other nurses. This course would enable the ENP to see the maximum number of patients but may be regarded as detracting from the holistic model of care which the ENP is able to provide (Woolwich, 1992).

A risk inherent in ENPs delegating nursing tasks to their colleagues is that they might come to be regarded as a substitute doctor or clinician's assistant rather than as a nurse specialist, with the ever increasing pressure to delegate some tasks to endeavour to relieve their workload. If this should be the case, would it be detrimental to overall patient care?

Lee (1988) stated that the interests of the patient should come before the throughput of the A and E department. Whilst improving the departmental throughput and efficiency and reducing overall waiting times may be in the interests of patients overall, a holistic approach to the care of individual patients would appear consistent with current nursing practice. If quality of care were to be regarded as the essential issue in introducing the ENP role, then a holistic approach without delegation might be easiest for ENPs when working within a community or hospital setting or with limited medical input, whilst in an existing A and E department where delegation of tasks to a variety of personnel is already practised, limited delegation in the pursuit of efficiency and quality might be a compromise solution.

Points for discussion

● Should ENPs carry out all treatments prescribed by themselves?

● Does delegation of tasks and treatments detract from holistic care?

● Is holistic care of patients really the prime concern of the ENP?

TRAINING REQUIRED

ENPs are required to utilize skills and techniques additional and different to those of other A and E nurses. It is understandably important that they be suitably qualified to perform these activities and that the qualification should be recognized as a guarantee of competence. Nurses should therefore undergo additional training to enable them to fulfil the ENP role and satisfactory completion of such training should be both documented and acknowledged (James and Pyrgos, 1989; Potter, 1990).

The ENP Special Interest Group (RCN, 1992) states clearly that the ENP is an A and E nurse with 'formal postbasic education recognized by the health authority and eventually by the statutory bodies as preparing her with the knowledge and skills required to fulfil the role' and recommends a framework for a syllabus of training based on four modules:

1. assessment and diagnosis;
2. treatment and prescribing;
3. communication skills;
4. health behaviour and prevention of injury and illness.

There is as yet, however, no nationally recognized training scheme for ENPs. Thus, individual departments are currently at liberty to decide for themselves if they require their ENPs to have undergone any formal postbasic education in the role. Should it be decided that such training is desirable, as suggested by numerous authors, then there are a variety of options possible.

The training needs of the ENP must be considered alongside the development of the role. If the role is seen as an integrated part of all A and E nursing (Burgess, 1992) it may be that the skills required are self-limiting. A very basic core of knowledge may be all that is required. However, if the role is seen as a clinical nurse specialist role, for dedicated ENPs with extensive experience in and knowledge of A and E nursing, a much more intensive training would be required.

There are currently several methods being employed to train ENPs. Nurses can be taken out of the clinical area and trained for a specific period. This may be a continuous period of time or done as part-day or day release inhouse by their own authorities. Alternatively nurses of suitable experience are trained on an individual basis. The training might take several months but the nurse comes to undertake the role once he or she feels able and comfortable with the experience attained. Another possible route that could be pursued is that prospective ENPs be seconded to intensive external courses of varying duration. The precise nature of such courses, including course content and duration, would have to be structured to accommodate the existing skills and expertise of those nurses attending.

A nationally agreed training programme?

One obvious disadvantage of any method that involves inhouse training is that such training does not automatically receive national acceptance and recognition. In order to avoid problems experienced by many nursing staff, not just those in A and E, in transferring acquired skills from a position in one hospital to another, a national qualification would seem desirable (Jones, 1986). Such a national qualification would in effect be a certification of abilities and training to a predetermined minimum level and hence these skills would be instantly recognized on the appointment of an ENP in a post anywhere in the UK. Thus an ENP trained nurse would be able to transfer and take up any ENP post in the country. Of course, there might still be the need to teach additional skills over and above those of this national certification scheme to cater for idiosyncrasies of given departments.

It has been advocated that the English National Board (ENB) provides a framework into which ENP training needs could be integrated. An ENB qualification could therefore provide a nationally recognized core of knowledge relating to the role. The precise mechanism of this is open to debate.

It has even been suggested that the existing ENB and A and E certfication (ENB 199) be expanded to incorporate ENP duties and responsibilities (Potter, 1990). The same author, however, goes on to point out that this might undermine the present qualification and decrease its suitability for those A and E nurses not seeking to work as ENPs for whom the ENB 199 is currently the foundation of their professional standing. However, with the integrated role, this may be a means for nurses interested in pursuing a career in A and E to obtain a basic first level knowledge that may be used in a limited ENP role.

For the development of a clinical nurse specialist role, however, this would not be adequate and a much more diverse and demanding training would be required. With the recent introduction of diplomas of nursing for all first level nurses it may be that courses to attain a minimum of diploma status may be the future of ENPs.

Clearly extensive further debate and research will be required to arrive at an ultimate solution satisfactory to proponents of each scheme. It should perhaps be borne in mind that the majority of those who train as ENPs in the USA are already highly trained nurses who obtain Masters degrees, having undergone a period of prolonged fulltime postgraduate studies to do so (Geolot, 1987). This would suggest that our transatlantic neighbours feel a hefty investment in time and money is required to adequately train their practitioners. It may well be that as the role develops in the UK, here too an increasingly rigorous and extensive training may need to be instituted.

Points for discussion

● What are the training needs of the ENP?

● What are the current training options for ENPs?

● Should there be a nationally agreed programme for ENP training?

● What form should such a programme take?

FINANCIAL IMPLICATIONS OF THE ROLE

ENP schemes have only been up and running in the UK since 1986 (Ramsden, 1986). A variety of different schemes have been implemented, involving in some cases the use of existing A and E staff rotating through the post as needs arise, in others the use of fulltime ENPs with no other A and E nursing commitments. As a result it is extremely difficult to quantify the costs and cost effectiveness of the implementation of ENP schemes in the United Kingdom.

Studies in the USA, where the role has existed far longer and where audit has long been routine, cannot be directly compared. The very different nature of health care financing in the USA, with private insurance schemes, different means of access to and different availability of back-up services (such as outpatient department appointments), means that only the broadest conclusions should be considered in weighing the implications for the UK. Broadly speaking, studies carried out in the USA would suggest that ENPs provide a substantially cheaper and equally effective alternative to more traditional emergency care provision (LeRoy, 1982; Sweet, 1986).

There is some suspicion that the British government favours the introduction of an ENP service on the assumption that nurses will provide a cheaper alternative to doctors (Warden, 1988). This highlights yet again the misconception of the role as being substitutive rather than complementary to that of the medical profession. It also overlooks the very real difficulties in evaluating the actual cost and savings accruing to health service financiers as a result of such ENP tasks as health promotion and prevention initiatives. These might result in additional use of services such as well women clinics at the GP surgery but cause fewer return visits to A and E departments.

Thus whilst people can freely make assumptions, there is as yet no reliable source of data to confirm or refute these. It will almost certainly be necessary to wait until many more schemes have been implemented and full audits carried out. Only then can the accuracy of any predictions as to the financial implications of the ENP role be commented upon. The cost implications surrounding the implementation of and training for ENP schemes beyond a basic first level is already recognized as a major consideration by those involved in the clinical area. It is clearly no cheap option but is perhaps 'an appropriate response' to the health needs of patients attending A and E departments throughout the United Kingdom (Walsh, 1989).

Points for discussion

● Can we learn from the USA experience regarding cost and cost effectiveness?

● What difficulties arise in evaluating cost effectiveness?

FUTURE DEVELOPMENTS

It is clear from the number of issues addressed that there are still many important decisions to be reached and strides to be made in establishing and further developing the ENP role. In order that these be the right ones for the nursing profession and for patients, it would be wise for all concerned with good practice to continue to air their views and also to listen to one another. In this way it ought to be possible to move forward with sensible, practical and agreeable formulae for the important future of this role. There is a great deal that ENPs can achieve within the confines of the A and E department and the increasing professional status and responsibility of the nursing profession can be exploited and enhanced by the role.

The development of the ENP role in the USA predates that in the UK by some decades. Thus it may be that future developments here will continue to mirror those that have already occurred in the USA. Whilst differences in the nature of health care provision in the UK and USA are quite significant, a brief examination of the way in which the USA ENP role is developing might provide a clue as to the future course of the profession in the UK.

In the USA, there continues to be rapid development and expansion of the role. There has been an increasing emphasis on the nursing theory, diagnosis, health promotion and counselling aspects of the role and a corresponding decrease in the training content of medical task orientated teaching (Geolot, 1987). The role of the ENP has expanded beyond its origins in the emergency room and now incorporates in addition the management of nursing duties housed in community clinics, senior citizens' complexes and on campuses

(Stainton *et al.*, 1989). As part of this role, ENPs have set up and run their own treatment rooms as well as arranging less urgent activities such as performing screening tests, physical examinations and health appraisals.

The latter activities cannot be seen as directly related to the current emergency service provision of ENPs in the UK; nonetheless, by this expansion of their responsibilities, ENPs in the USA are now providing patients with a real alternative to their general medical practitioner as well as to the hospital based emergency room. Meanwhile, nurse practitioners within the hospital environment continue to function so successfully that the use of ENPs has been advocated as a substitute for medical staff in residency programmes (Silver and McAtee, 1988).

New Zealand is a country which mirrors the traditions, training and practice of our own UK nursing profession. There, nurses are also seeking changes to their working practice. They are making representations to government bodies at present, looking at the legal implications of independent nurse practitioners working in a self-employed capacity outside their National Health Service. Nurses are seeking independence from hospitals, setting themselves up as self-employed, autonomous practitioners with 'a well-defined and recognized area of responsibility' (Messervy, 1991). Naturally this process 'requires courage and determination, it is a movement which has raised curiosity, concern, fear and anger amongst some sectors of the health care service' (Hawkins, 1989).

The way forward for UK ENPs

The establishment and development of the ENP role in the UK is not yet so far along such an independent route. Indeed, it remains to be seen whether such expansion of the role is generally desired. It may be that in the UK the nursing profession will be able to develop a model of practice unique to our environment. The choice of future is not yet decided – the role is in the process of evolution (Burgess, 1992) and it is up to nurses and ENPs to decide what future they want for the role and in what directions it will develop. They must then be the ones to lobby for that future.

Points for discussion

● What has been happening in the USA?

● Is the experience of New Zealand a guide to the future of ENPs in the UK or is an alternative approach required?

REFERENCES

Aiken, L. (1982) *Nursing in the 1980s: Crises, Opportunities, Challenges,* J.B. Lippincott, Philadelphia, pp. 295–314.

Andrews, S. (1988) An expert in practice. *Nursing Times,* **84**(26), 31–3.

Beachley, M. and Snow, S. (1988) Developing trauma care systems. The trauma nurse coordinator. *Journal of Nursing Administration,* **18**(7/8), 34–42.

Becker, K., Zaiken, H. and Wilcox, P. (1989) A nurse practitioner's job description. *Nursing Management,* **20**(6), 42–4.

Beloff, J. and Paris, H. (1967) Outpatient services. *American Hospital Association Journal,* **41**(4), 143.

Blythin, P. (1988a) Triage in the UK. *Nursing,* **3**(31), 16–20.

Blythin, P. (1988b) Triage documentation. *Nursing,* **3**(32), 32–4.

Bowling, A. (1987) Practice nurses: the future role. *Nursing Times,* **83**(17), 31–3.

Burgess, K. (1992) A dynamic role that improves the service. *Professional Nurse,* **7**(5), 301–3.

Cliff, K.S. (1974) Accident and emergency care: the role of the nurses. *Nursing Times,* **70**(38), 1448–9.

Council for Professions Supplementary to Medicine (1989) *Radiographers Board Statement of Conduct,* CPSM, London.

Cumberlege, J. (1986) *Neighbourhood Nursing: A Focus for Care.* Report of the Community Nursing Review (The Cumberlege Report), DHSS/HMSO, London.

Department of Health (1991) *The Patients Charter,* HMSO, London.

Fagin, C.M. (1982) Nursing as an alternative to high cost care. *American Journal of Nursing,* **82**(1), 56–60.

Fawcett-Henesy, A. (1990) Setting the scene for revolution. *Nursing Standard,* **4**(21), 35.

Geolot, D. (1987) Nurse practitioner education: observations from a national perspective. *Nursing Outlook,* **35**(3), 132–5.

Geolot, D., Alongis, S. and Edlich, R.F. (1977) Emergency nurse practitioners: an answer to an emergency room crisis in rural hospitals. *Journal of the American College of Emergency Physicians,* **6**(8), 355–7.

Gould, D. (1988) Opportunities for the accident and emergency nurse. *Nursing,* **3**(31), 24–6.

Hawkins, L. (1989) *Nurses Who See Themselves as Independent Practitioners,* New Zealand Nurses Association Research Paper, unpublished.

Head, S. (1988) The new pioneers. *Nursing Times,* **84**(26), 27–8.

James, M.R. and Pyrgos, N. (1989) Nurse practitioners in the accident and emergency department. *Archives of Emergency Medicine,* **6**(4), 241–6.

Jones, G. (1986) Accident and emergecy . . . behind the times. *Nursing Times,* **82**(42), 30–3.

Jones, G. (1988) Top priority. *Nursing Standard,* **3**(7), 28–9.

La Plant, L.J. and O'Bannol, F.V. (1987) Nurse practitioners – prescribing recommendations. *Nurse Practitioner,* **12**(4), 52–3, 57–8.

Lee, M. (1988) The nurse practitioner in the A&E department: a feasible way forward. *Emergency Nurse,* **3**(1), 2–3.

LeRoy, L. (1982) The cost effectiveness of nurse practitioners, in *Nursing in the 1980s,* (ed. L. Aiken), J.B. Lippincott, Philadelphia.

Lewis, B.R. and Bradbury, Y. (1982) The role of the nursing profession in hospital accident and emergency departments. *Journal of Advanced Nursing,* **7**, 211–21.

Lewis, C.E. and Resnick, B.A. (1967) Nurse clinics and progressive ambulatory patient care. *New England Journal of Medicine,* **277**, 1236–41.

Mallett, J. and Woolwich, C. (1990) Triage in A&E departments. *Journal of Advanced Nursing*, **15**(12), 1443–5.

Markham, G. (1988) Special cases. *Nursing Times*, **84**(2), 29–30.

Messervy, L. (1991) *The Rise of the Independent Practitioner*, unpublished case study.

Milward, P. (1990) Prescribing dressings. *Journal of District Nursing*, **5**, 5–6.

Pearson, A. (1983) *The Clinical Nursing Unit*, Heinemann, London.

Potter, T. (1990) A real way forward in A&E. *Professional Nurse*, **5**(11), 586–8.

Ramsden, S. (1986) *Nurse Practitioner Evaluation Report on Trial Period*, Barking, Havering and Brentwood Health Authority, Essex.

Rice, T. (1989) Thames RHA focus. *Nursing Standard*, **3**(45), 45.

Royal College of Nursing (1992) *Report of Special Interest Group on Accident and Emergency Nurse Practitioners*, RCN, London.

Salkever, D.S., Skinner, E.A. and Steinwachs, D.M. (1982) Episode-based efficiency comparisons for physicians and nurse practitioners. *Medical Care*, **20**(2), 143–53.

Salvage, J. (1990) The nurse practitioner – everybody's relative but nobody's baby. *Nursing Standard*, **4**(21), 49–50.

Silver, H.K. and McAtee, P. (1988) Should nurses substitute for house staff? *American Journal of Nursing*, **86**(12), 1671–3.

Simon, P. (1992) No doctor in the house. *Nursing Times*, **88**(8), 28.

Sox, H.C. Jr (1979) Quality of patient care by nurse practitioners and physician's assistants – a ten year study. *Annals of International Medicine*, **9**(3), 459–68.

Spitzer, W.O., Sackett, D.L. and Sibley, J.C. (1974) The Burlington randomized trial of the nurse practitioner. *New England Journal of Medicine*, **290**, 251–6.

Stainton, M.C., Rankin, J.A. and Calkin, J.D. (1989) The development of a practising nursing faculty. *Journal of Advanced Nursing*, **14**(1), 20–6.

Stilwell, B. (1982) The nurse practitioner at work in primary care. *Nursing Times*, **78**(17), 1796–803.

Sweet, J.B. (1986) The cost effectiveness of nurse practitioners. *Nursing Economics*, **4**(4), 190–3.

Tettersall, M. (1988) Defining the boundaries. *Nursing Standard*, **3**(7), 22–3.

Tooley, S. and Field, P.A. (1985) Parents' perception of care. *Nursing Mirror*, **161**(19), 38–40.

United Kingdom Central Council (1992) *Scope of Professional Practice*, UKCC, London.

Walker, M.L. (1986) The clinical nurse specialist as a consultant. *Nursing Management*, **17**(5), 61.

Walsh, M. (1989) The accident and emergency department and the nurse practitioner. *Nursing Standard*, **4**(11), 34–6.

Warden, J. (1988) The rise of the nurse practitioner. *British Medical Journal*, **296**, 1478–9.

Widhalm, S.A. and Anderson, L.A. (1982) Emergency nurse practitioners: motivators, barriers and autonomy in role performance. *Journal of Emergency Nursing*, **8**(2), 67–74.

Woolwich, C. (1992) A wider frame of reference. *Nursing Times*, **88**(46), 34–6.

CHAPTER 2

Liaison psychiatry in A and E

S.P. Edgeley and D.W. Rowell

INTRODUCTION

Psychiatric liaison is a developing area of A and E work yet many nurses find it difficult to deal with those with a mental health problem seeking the services of an A and E department. There are various reasons for this, some of which may be related to the lack of preparation of nurses to care for those with a mental health problem, lack of facilities and an inappropriate environment. The last two reasons border on the 'inappropriate attender' debate which readers may wish to develop from information introduced in this chapter.

This chapter concentrates upon mental health problems only. It does not examine the needs of those who have physical disabilities although it is acknowledged that this area of need does require examination in A and E. Whilst working through this chapter, the reader is asked to focus upon their beliefs relating to the use of A and E services by the mentally ill. In addition, readers should consider the appropriateness of the A and E environment, the number of persons with mental health problems being seen in any one A and E department and how various authorities liaise to provide a service for those with mental health problems. As with other chapters in the book, this chapter does not hold any answers for the reader and the reader is expected to challenge ideas and standpoints put forward. The chapter is organized to promote readers' questioning of their own knowledge and understanding of how care is provided for the person with a mental health problem. This is done by considering a number of mental health conditions which are then handed over to the reader to consider within their own area of practice via the use of discussion points. Points for discussion are used in conjunction with suggestions for discussion. Both provide a guide to the questioning of information and ideas put forward. It is expected that the reader will add extra questions to those in the text.

Anecdotes are used within the chapter to illustrate points made. In addition the use of one particular psychiatric liaison service is introduced by the contributors to show organization and management of such a service. It is expected that this will provide a basis upon which other local mental health services can be examined. In addition the reader is asked to consider a nationally provided service and its potential relationship with the A and E service.

References at the end of the chapter should provide a starting point for further reading about points put forward in the text.

The introduction of the 1959 Mental Health Act (DHSS, 1959) promoted the so-called 'open door policy' which then developed in all the psychiatric institutions. Since 1959, empirically attitudes and strongly held views about the mentally ill have begun to change towards being more positive.

The aims of emergency psychiatric practice are relatively rapid evaluation, containment and referral to the appropriate agency for further care (Gerson and Bassuk, 1980). Although both the Accident and Emergency team and the liaison psychiatric team have the same objective, the patient is often lost in the maelstrom of bureaucracy and other priorities in the department. Despite the positive development of triage (Dunn and Fernando, 1989), many patients are never seen.

Points for discussion

- Although it may be suggested that generally, attitudes toward the mentally ill are more positive, is this true of the Accident and Emergency department?

- New legislation has heralded the development of a more appropriate service for both the mentally ill and those people with psychological problems (DoH, 1992). However, it may be interesting to discover whether the view that those who deliberately self-harm are seen as mentally ill is held throughout the country or whether Accident and Emergency teams believe that such a view is appropriate at the 'sharp end' of acute care?

The 1962 Hospital Plan (DHSS, 1962) recommended the widespread establishment of psychiatric services based in district general hospitals and the closure of many of the old mental hospitals, many of which had attracted considerable criticism. There is no doubt that the pendulum has swung back towards reintegrating psychiatry within medicine. This aspect of psychiatry has come to be known as liaison psychiatry, an imperfect term but one which emphasizes the links which psychiatry has developed with other specialities.

Dunn and Fernando (1989) examined the A and E records at a London hospital and found that during a six month period, 464 patients were judged primarily to have a 'psychiatric' disorder. These constituted 2% of all attendants to the A and E department, a figure similar to that previously reported by Anstee (1972). One psychiatrist saw 52% of these patients and 36% were admitted to hospital. Amongst the diagnostic categories described, patients with alcohol related problems received the least intervention.

Based on current figures in Leicester (MHSU, 1992) the 2% figure of 1972 has risen and deliberate self-harm now accounts for 9% of all attendants to A and E. Alarming figures when balanced against the resources offered to this client group in the A and E department.

Despite government legislation, such as *The Health of the Nation* (DoH, 1992) and *The Patients Charter* (DoH, 1991), there is still a need for positive changes in both attitudes and investments in the care of the mentally ill and those who are psychologically ill. Martin (1984) has shown that a major cause of inertia and suboptimal performance in the mental health care arena is related to self-interested and destructive professional rivalries. Rather than genuinely addressing the problems of how best to serve those consumers most in need, some members of the care providing groups appear to have been more concerned to pursue their own interests, existing employment patterns and power relationships.

DELIBERATE SELF-HARM

During the 1960s Accident and Emergency departments throughout the country saw a massive increase in the number of people deliberately self-harming either by an overdose of tablets or by self-injury. One of the reasons for such an increase at this time was the introduction of the Suicide Act of 1961 (Hawton and Catalan, 1987), by which attempted suicide ceased to be a criminal act.

Recent figures (Hawton and Catalan, 1987) show that some 100 000 deliberate self-harm referrals are made to Accident and Emergency departments each year. It is the single most common reason for hospital admission for women, second only to that of heart disease for men. These figures only reflect the numbers that present: many people do not seek treatment and others leave the Accident and Emergency department prior to seeing a doctor. Overall it has been estimated that only one in four seeks medical contact using hospital or general practitioners.

Due to the alarming incidence of deliberate self-harm each year, Accident and Emergency guidelines for the management of this client group were published (DHSS/Royal College of Psychiatrists, 1984). These recommended that every district health authority should make arrangements for the management of persons following deliberate self-harm and should have a clearly laid down policy. It also emphasized the need for good liaison between the agencies involved in the community and hospital based services.

Such recommendations have influenced the setting up of deliberate self-harm services throughout the country, which include psychiatrists, specialist nurses and social workers. Many come under the umbrella of the liaison psychiatric services. Catalan *et al.* (1980) concluded that there were no major differences between the initial assessment carried out by a nurse or a doctor on a patient who had deliberately self-harmed, where the nurse was a member of a team which had a psychiatrist available for consultation and supervision.

These services have had great influences upon A and E departments decreasing the amount of time that someone has to wait to be assessed. One of the key improvements was to have a member of the deliberate self-harm team on site, specially skilled to assess risk factors, suicide intent, mental state examination and to give specific guidelines on the person's management and aftercare.

A number of services around the country have a network of resources available, some offering a follow-up service for specific therapies, for example crisis intervention and problem solving approaches. It also allows for the retuning of attitudes regarding deliberate self-harm, by working alongside the A and E nurses using a collaborative model (Hicks, 1989), with a specific focus on addressing the educational needs of the carers.

Often it is stated that people who deliberately self-harm only do it for attention. In some cases this may be true but it can be seen as a conscious or unconscious manipulation to change their environment to regain control. It is often used as a mechanism for coping, with little intent to die, and the act is usually spontaneous and in response to current life stresses. However, there is a proportion of people who genuinely wish they had succeeded. These are generally known as failed suicides.

Specific risk factors that influence the assessment of a person following deliberate self-harm are listed below:

1. Prevalence of suicide in males;
2. Unemployed/retired;
3. Widowed/separated/divorced;
4. Physical illness;
5. Social environment/isolation;

6. Previous DSH;
7. Family history of suicide;
8. Drug/alcohol dependency;
9. Method of suicide/suicide note;
10. Mental health problem.

Triage

Triage is a system of sorting patients according to priority (Grose, 1988). As a consequence of this role the nurse is the first carer to address the patient's needs. It is at triage that most people feel that there needs to be some change. Many would argue that a specialized nurse should intervene, although clearly such a person would be overwhelmed with referrals for every disturbed individual that presents to A and E. In one area within the Trent region, each deliberate self-harm client is treated with the same priority as a head injury.

Eighteen percent of people who deliberately self-harm leave the A and E department as a direct result of having to wait for long periods of time, even though their crisis may not have been resolved (MHSU, 1992). Clearly supervision is an issue, often rectified by providing a specific area in which the patients can be monitored. Alternatively the simple method of supplying a courtesy letter identifying contact agencies if A and E is too busy acts effectively to minimize the risk to those who leave prior to assessment and/or intervention.

A number of patients have found it difficult to discuss their problems. This is not because of lack of rapport, a breakdown in communication or lack of trust, but because of the lack of privacy, space and time to reflect. A busy A and E department does not lend itself to people who need to discuss their psychological problems. People often feel that they will be rejected, reprimanded, belittled or stereotyped.

It is easy to identify problems in the way we care for people with this presentation, but it is less easy to find ways in which they can be resolved. The key route has to be via education of nurses and carers, thereby creating a better understanding. This involves not just attending a course periodically, but the development of skills on a continuous basis by the allocation of A and E nurses for a fixed period in which they are responsible directly for all deliberate self-harm patients when on duty. They will have a better understanding via such involvement of the need for collaboration with the nurse specialist of the deliberate self-harm team.

Points for discussion

● It may be asked how can someone who has deliberately self-harmed have priority over acute physical trauma? You need to take into consideration the lack of challenge to traditional attitudes, as well as the emphasis upon skill and knowledge base of the individual nurse who is caring for this complex and sometimes 'difficult' human being.

● Can the setting up of a liaison team be seen as an effective tool in delivering the most effective care in the treatment of these patients? Clearly in this text suggestions are made that education and collaboration in expert intervention is going some way to achieve this. Or is this going to be a major threat to the required eclectic skills of the A and E nurse?

● Taking into consideration environmental needs, in what way do you feel that changes could be carried out to improve the care and influence the reduction of associated trauma? When addressing this, consider the level of observation required and achievable in the A and E department today.

Legislation (DHSS, 1983) does not permit the holding of a patient unless they are seen as mentally ill or they are within a life-threatening situation. Even within these circumstances people are allowed to go after assessment due to the governing regulations of the Mental Health Act 1983. The act of deliberate self-harm is the individual's own responsibility and right and does not always constitute a mental illness. The nurse may find this difficult to accept so it is important to recognize the need for good communication and trust between the A and E nurses and the liaison psychiatric team to ease the anxieties expressed.

Points for discussion

● Consider the influence of the Mental Health Act 1983 in the assessment of a patient and the probable outcome.

AFFECTIVE DISORDERS

Depression has been described as the common cold of psychiatry. The term encompasses a range of states, from near normal moods of sadness to clinical conditions of life-threatening seriousness (Brown, 1989). Morbid depression is associated not only with suicide but also with problems such as child neglect and abuse. It is a state of mind characterized by loss of an individual's self-worth and his/her ability to enjoy life (Brown, 1989).

The psychological symptoms of depression are widely described in texts, yet in a busy A and E department such symptoms of sadness, worthlessness, paranoia and biological symptomatology, amongst many others (Lader, 1981), are so easily missed.

Point for discussion

● Perhaps the reason is that such symptoms are so evident in all forms of trauma and associated emotional distress that the A and E nurse becomes immune to such presentations. Also, often the patients themselves do not disclose their feelings. More appropriately, the answer has to be sought in the mechanism of communication, environment, human responses, attitudes and the wish to elicit such information when the individual is not physically traumatized.

The radical change brought about by the Children Act (DoH, 1989) and the need to serve children on a more suitable level have led A and E departments to become more aware of such matters as environment, communication and attitudes when catering for the needs of the child brought into A and E. Such changes took time and a more proactive approach, rather than allowing nurses to feel threatened when questioned about their approach to and care of children.

Attempting to communicate with a depressed person on a level that engages a sense of warmth, trust, empathy and understanding is complex. If the environment is more receptive to these emotions, chances of engagement are increased by 30%. There should be privacy, comfort, appropriate lighting, room temperature and wall colouring. These may all be absent in some A and E departments.

Eye contact and a non-verbal approach are so important and in many cases the individual is lost as a result of the breakdown of these two basic principles. When one talks, tone, clarity and an air of wanting to listen are important but the most vital component is time. The use of open or closed questioning is seen as a skill, yet someone who shows empathy and has time to listen can often deduce information not attained in a formal interview.

Attitudes towards the person who is depressed are best illustrated by feedback given by a patient who presented herself at A and E. She felt that the carers wanted to find out what was wrong physically and when told there was nothing, they became hostile and belligerent and uninterested in attempting to understand what her needs were. She stated that she felt like a second class citizen and was looked upon as a nuisance when she informed them that she wanted help because of feeling desperate and depressed. It is hard to believe that such an attitude could be taken in the 1990s. Interestingly, this woman was a nurse herself.

A and E culture and attitudes are changing with the investment in education and the influence of liaison psychiatry, but the environment still remains poor when addressing the needs of those with mental health problems.

Points for discussion

● The influence of A and E culture, attitudes, application of appropriate skills and seeing the person as an individual are all important aspects of care. Where does the high risk group of depressed people come in the rating of need?

The number of people coming through A and E who are formally depressed is low (Atha *et al.*, 1989). However, there are increasing numbers of those who are depressed or suffering with anxiety attributed to trauma, physical illness or a reactive state such as profound grief. The liaison psychiatric team has an increasing role in catering for the needs of these client groups within the A and E department. The emphasis on the collaborative model has never been greater.

COLLABORATIVE MODEL

The collaborative model has been used effectively across Europe and America. Jane Dunn (1989) applied the model within the emergency room of a hospital in Illinois, where there was key collaboration between the psychiatric services and emergency room team.

Effectively, the liaison nurse specialist (provider) has a partnership with the organizational service (user) with both parties having specific contributions:

Liaison Nurse Specialist	A and E Staff
Support	Essential information
Expert knowledge	Knowledge
Skills	Skills
Objectivity	Resources

(Dunn, 1989)

Consequently the client receives the optimum care they require from both a physical and psychological point of view.

Point for discussion

● Is this the most appropriate model to apply when addressing the psychological needs of patients within the A and E department or should we be focusing on the skill and knowledge base of the A and E nurse rather than the collaboration with the specialist team?

LIFE PROBLEMS

Life problems such as marital discord, sexual and physical abuse, social isolation including unemployment, homelessness, financial problems and mental health problems of old age may all act as instigators of formal or adjustment disorders that may present in an A and E department. All of these may appear superficial but require careful and effective management and intervention.

The psychiatry of old age is a specialist area. The need for specific collaboration between psychiatric liaison, A and E and elderly care teams has to be addressed within the A and E department if better service is to be promoted and offered to the ageing population.

VICTIMS OF VIOLENCE

Victims of violence are frequent visitors to the A and E department. Empirical evidence suggests that not all nurses in A and E and in other settings can cope. In order to achieve this one must be aware of what constitutes violence. Webster (1977) defined violence as an act marked by extreme force, a sudden intense activity to the point of loss of one's self control. Victims of this act can be categorized into five main groups:

1. physical violence to the person;
2. psychological violence;
3. material violence;
4. social violence;
5. sexual violence.

(Stuart and Sundeen, 1983)

Victims of violence are usually female and the aggressor is usually known to them (Lloyd, 1991). They are usually in crisis obscured by psychological defences and reactions, including anger, anxiety, lowering of mood, tearfulness and despair. In the long term insomnia with early morning waking, recurring dreams and 'flashbacks' of the assault are common. These symptoms are characteristic of post-traumatic stress (Turnquist *et al.*, 1988), as well as a depressive illness. It is easy to understand why it is often believed that such a presentation constitutes a mental illness. However the presentation should be recognized as an adjustment process in most instances and not a mental illness.

Responses need to be immediate. Being allowed to discuss the event will reduce initial anxieties and fear. The person also needs to be allowed to express the way he or she feels. In addition, environmental issues have to be addressed to enable the victim to feel safe, encouraging self-disclosure of confidential issues related to the event. It is sometimes necessary that other agencies such as rape crisis may have to be involved. Accident and Emergency policies for such circumstances should be clear in establishing criteria for access to other agencies.

Although it is clear that the liaison psychiatric nurses should have the skills to address the needs of the individual, in most instances the outside specialist agencies can take more of a primary role, particularly if it is believed that the presentation does not constitute a psychiatric illness. Alternatively, it may be recognized that the individual may become so seriously ill that the liaison team would be required to work on a consultation basis in collaboration with the outside agency and the A and E team. An important role for the liaison psychiatric nurse is in education, support and developing the necessary skills within A and E nurses to meet such clients. The liaison psychiatric nurse can also work as a coordinator alongside A and E nurses in developing A and E nurses' skills and approaches in relation to people with mental health problems.

The liaison psychiatric service has also begun to act, at the request of the voluntary sector, in a supervisory role to counsellors in the A and E department. Although valuable to both parties, this has a depleting effect on the liaison psychiatric service and provokes the question of whether individual health authorities should be addressing the needs of various client groups. Overall mental health related evaluations and audits of interventions of groups of carers in A and E are required.

It is interesting to note that to date there has been no valuable audit of psychiatric intervention within the A and E department. We are sure that such a process would highlight alarming evidence when addressing appropriate standards of care.

Points for discussion

- It is necessary to address the resource implication for victims of violence, especially if we are to accept that environment has a major role in regard to catering for individual needs.

- It is suggested that this client group does not have a mental illness. How can someone distinguish where the line of diagnosis lies when the problems become indicative of a mental illness and yet are classified as part of an adjustment reaction?

- An audit to quantify and qualify indivdual needs appears to be required. How much value would a separate facility, away from the A and E department, have for this client group?

ORGANIC PRESENTATIONS

One of the most disturbing presentations is that of individuals with disorders of either perception or thought, attributed to a number of problems associated with organic or psychotic disorders or substance abuse, with the possibility of violence to self or others.

Hallucinations involving any of the five senses bring about a distortion of reality and as a consequence the individual feels a sense of lack of control, so that any intervention may be seen as hostile, intimidating or anxiety provoking. The individual's fears are difficult to determine but the distress caused can be fatal. The lack of insight creates a situation that is difficult to control and which can give rise to frustration on the part of the carers. This may bring about negative management decisions which are destructive to the individual in the A and E department.

Thought disturbances may induce so much distress at the point of crisis that management can be next to non-existent without the use of chemotherapy. Although this may give the impression that the patient is a major problem, he or she is likely to be more distressed within themselves than with others.

Once again environment plays a major role in the care of such people and emphasis should be placed on the safety aspects (Lloyd, 1991). Arguments are made that an intensive care facility for the psychiatrically ill is required in close proximity to the A and E department. In a number of areas the liaison psychiatric ward is used as such a facility, although little evidence has been put forward to support this. Indeed, the concept of a psychiatric intensive care unit (PICU) has now been recognized as being the most effective approach, tailoring skilled approaches and environment to the needs of this client group. It remains to be seen whether this facility will be extended for direct referrals from A and E.

Point for discussion

● With the associated trauma and intensity of the problem, is this not the most classic indication for psychiatric emergency care? How effectively can the current A and E service cater for these individuals' needs?

ALCOHOL AND DRUG DEPENDENCY

Alcohol and drug dependency are often seen as a consequence of modern day society, a statement that probably acts as an excuse for many and an irritant to others. Within psychiatry many argue that neither constitutes a mental illness.

The World Health Organization (1977) defines 'alcoholics' as excessive drinkers whose dependence on alcohol has attained such a degree that it causes a notable mental disturbance or an interference with their body and mental health, their interpersonal relations and their social and economic functions. A similar description could be applied to drug abuse.

Patients attending A and E departments because of alcohol abuse are generally referred to the local alcohol counselling service or hospital based treatment unit, dependent upon the severity of presentation. This procedure can be said to be the same for drug abuse. In both cases the physical treatment process can be hampered by a number of neurological problems or self-neglect. Indeed a large number of people may have to sleep overnight in an A and E department to allow a more accurate assessment of their physical, psychological and social needs the next day.

There are numerous texts that describe the associated syndromes in both areas of abuse (Lockhart *et al.*, 1986; Quinn and Johnson, 1976). However there is clear evidence that patients with alcohol problems receive the least intervention (Anstee, 1972).

Despite evidence to suggest that there has been an increase in the number of referrals for help with alcohol or drug dependency over the last 20 years, this client group still remains the one with the least intervention (MHSU, 1991a).

Hawton's work (1989) in Oxford on the association of alcoholism with deliberate self-harm showed that of 7006 people assessed, 7.9% received a diagnosis of 'alcoholism', this diagnosis being made for more males than females.

The incidence of alcohol related problems in the A and E department is partly due to the major role that alcohol plays in industrial, domestic and road traffic accidents. Glynn and O'Neill (1974) found that 26% of patients admitted to the A and E department at night were 'inebriated' but most were allowed home without follow-up when sober. In another study (Holt, 1980) 24% of those patients attending A and E were admitted on the basis of alcohol related circumstances. Forty per cent had consumed alcohol before arrival in A and E and 32% had a blood alcohol concentration that exceeded the legal limit for driving a motor vehicle. Recent consumption was identified in patients with impaired levels of consciousness. Yates *et al.* (1987) showed that blood alcohol levels were especially high in patients following assaults and road traffic accidents and in those brought in by the police.

Despite having alcohol services to support the main psychiatric services, it is suggested that there are not enough resources to allow direct intervention from the counselling service to the A and E department or psychiatric liaison service. In the majority of cases patients are either referred on or refer themselves. It is debatable whether this is the most effective way of helping people with such a dependency.

The referral of patients with drug dependency is extremely low and generally the reason for a referral for mental health assessment is given as 'deliberate self-harm'. It is recognized that management of those clients choosing alcohol and drugs is difficult with regard to physical care. However, recorded admission of such patients is only done in extreme cases of drug induced psychosis (management previously discussed in the text). Recent comparisons (MHSU, 1991b) of Leicester's liaison psychiatric services and the liaison consultation service in Vu, Amsterdam, showed that the incidence of deliberate self-harm related to drug dependency was low in both areas, despite the high incidence of drug dependency in Amsterdam. Leicestershire and Amsterdam have a similar population breakdown, specifically in relation to ethnicity. It is interesting to note that there is a high incidence of drug related deliberate self-harm of British citizens visiting Amsterdam, compared to other nationalities.

Points for discussion

- Considering the problems related to alcohol and drug abuse, what direct specialized resources are available to support the A and E team in the management of persons presenting with alcohol and/or drug abuse?

- Current reviews of both the alcohol and drug services have taken place to evaluate the service, in line with recommendations to offer a better service. However, can such reviews meet the need that is being suggested, when we address the relationship of this type of abuse with other referrals to the A and E department?

CONCLUSION

Fear of mental illness, and those who suffer with it, is not simply related to the suspicion that all those who are psychiatrically disturbed are a danger to others. The roots lie also in the challenge that mental illness may present to established interpretations of reality and the underlying threat that contact with such distress may somehow unmask previously repressed conflicts in the minds of 'normal people'. In addition to the stigma that all groups of disabled people have in the past had to suffer, individuals with psychiatric conditions have encountered rejection stemming from, in a sense, the desire of those around them to avoid contagion.

This is still reflected in some of today's debates about community care, psychotropic medication and the influence of society on the treatment of the mentally ill, all of which affects the care delivery within an A and E department.

The *Health of the Nation* government report (DoH, 1992) isolated those attempting deliberate self-harm as the largest patient group treated for mental health problems in the A and E department. Unfortunately it is society that will have to decide whether attitudes are to change despite the positive approach of legislation and the trend inspired by government to positively acknowledge the mentally ill. Perhaps if some of the attitudes of those with A and E departments could be challenged, people with mental health problems might get the service they deserve.

It is true that the level of expertise and support both in education and direct, effective nursing care needs a boost. However, this cannot effectively work until the key carers are receptive and willing to change the routines and approaches that have remained the same for many years. With the input of liaison psychiatry and the support of active community mental health teams, it is hoped that the established professional carers have the chance to make the change a reality.

It is understandable that nurses orientated to physical care needs have the attitude that mental illness is 'not my problem', an attitude predominantly due to the lack of understanding and skill to help the individual. It is necessary to address the education of general nursing and the developing Project 2000 nursing syllabus in order to increase the profile of psychiatric emergencies, rather than the established courses which look at all aspects of mental health in a small amount of time. Continuing education will play its role in changing attitudes, but many argue that it skates over the surface of what is required. It may be interesting to know what level of education is required to change attitudes and approaches to psychiatric emergencies, which encompass the physical and psychological needs of, for example, the self-harm patient.

The active involvement of nurses from the liaison psychiatric team in the A and E department should influence the care given to patients with psychological or psychiatric problems, both directly or in conjunction with the nurses in A and E. For this, investment in a training programme is required with the psychiatric and A and E nurses acting as change agents, the outcome of which should be greater emphasis on positive care delivery.

It is argued that there needs to be an investment of fulltime registered mental nurses within the A and E department (Sheenham 1991); as mentioned earlier, such involvement could have serious implications for practice, especially since such a role would probably encompass restraining and diffusing violent acts. Many prefer the active involvement of nurses from the liaison psychiatric team, with a wider range of experience, more support resources and a level of expertise that enables the nurse to tackle issues that may require a continuity of care and a greater level of accountability and responsibility.

It is true that the clinical nurse specialist role in liaison psychiatry, applicable to the A and E department, has not been sufficiently evaluated with regard to its effectiveness. However, the role is still in its infancy. The seconding of qualified A and E nurses to the liaison psychiatric team is seen as a viable approach to support the professional development of the nurse as well as enhancing the care given to the patient who has a mental health problem.

Reference to the collaborative model has been made in this text, predominantly due to the need for this to be recognized as an effective tool to develop the care of the person with a mental health problem. One of the major goals has to be forging better communication links and working together to support both levels of expertise. This still remains poor in a number of A and E departments, with the feeling that practice is being questioned, and therefore practice is carried out in isolation rather than together for the betterment of the patient.

Environmental issues are said to be harder to address, predominantly due to cost, despite the difficulty of differentiating between the costing of all the other aspects discussed and the environmental needs. The drive to change to a more personal, private and conducive environment remains low despite the empirical evidence of its link to the loss of patients, sometimes with fatal consequences.

It is said that the best judge of the service is the patient; he or she will give a more precise opinion than any of the professionals involved. A lot of the arguments put forward have much so-called 'weight' but none more than the statement of a patient saying, 'I just want to be treated like everyone else, with the chance to get better, with the dignity and respect that I deserve'. A powerful thought when determining priorities.

REFERENCES

Anstee, B.H. (1972) Psychiatry in the casualty department. *British Journal of Psychiatry*, **120**, 625–9.

Atha, C., Salkorsis, P. and Storer, D. (1989) Problem solving treatment. *Nursing Times*, **85**(17), 45–7.

Brown, G.W. (1989) *Social Origins of Depression*, Tavistock, London.

Catalan, J., Marsack, P., Hawton, K.E. *et al.* (1980) Comparison of doctors and nurses in the assessment of deliberate self-poisoning patients. *Psychological Medicine*, **10**, 483–91.

Department of Health (1989) *Children Act*, HMSO, London.

Department of Health (1991) *Patients Charter*, HMSO, London.

Department of Health (1992) *Health of the Nation*, HMSO, London.

Department of Health and Social Security (1959) *Mental Health Act*, HMSO, London.

Department of Health and Social Security (1962) *Hospital Plan*, HMSO, London.

Department of Health and Social Security (1983) *Mental Health Act*, HMSO, London.

DHSS/Royal College of Psychiatrists (1984) *Guidelines on the Management of Deliberate Self-Harm*, HMSO, London.

Dunn, J. (1989) Psychiatric interventions in the community emergency room. *Journal of Nursing Administration*, **19**(10), 36–40.

Dunn, J. and Fernando, R. (1989) Psychiatric presentation to an accident and emergency department. *Psychiatric Bulletin*, **13**, 672–4.

Gerson, S. and Bassuk, E. (1980) Psychiatric emergencies – an overview. *American Journal of Psychiatry*, **137**, 1–11.

Glynn, J. and O'Neill, F. (1974) Social interventions with intoxicated patients seen in accident and emergency. *Journal of the Irish Medical Association*, **67**, 40–2.

Grose, A. (1988) Triage in accident and emergency. *Professional Nurse*, **6**, 21–6.

Hawton, K. (1989) Alcohol and alcohol attempted suicide. *Alcohol and Alcoholism*, **24**(19), 3–9.

Hawton, K. and Catalan, J. (1987) *Attempted Suicide*, Oxford University Press, Oxford.

Hicks, S. (1989) The psychiatric nurse in liaison psychiatry. *Australian and New Zealand Journal of Psychiatry*, **23**, 89–96.

Holt, S. (1980) Alcohol and the emergency services. *British Medical Journal*, **281**, 638–40.

Lader, M.H. (1981) *Focus on Depression*, Bencard, London.

Lloyd, G. (1991) Screening problem drinkers among medical inpatients, in *Textbook of General Hospital Psychiatry*, (ed. G.G. Lloyd), Churchill Livingstone, Edinburgh, pp. 355–9.

Lockhart, S.P., Carter, Y.H., Staffen, A.M. *et al.* (1986) Detecting alcohol consumption. *Journal of the Royal Society of Medicine*, **79**, 136–9.

Martin, F.M. (1984) *Between the Acts: Community Mental Health Services*, Nuffield Provincial, Hospital Trust, London.

MHSU (1991a) *Alcohol Services Annual Report*, MHSU, Leicester.

MHSU (1991b) *European Exchange Scheme*, MHSU, Leicester.

MHSU (1992) *Mental Health Services Unit Annual Report*, MHSU, Leicester.

Quinn, M.A. and Johnson, H.V. (1976) Alcohol problems in acute medical admissions. *Health Bulletin*, **34**, 253–6.

Sheenham, A. (1991) RMNs have a part to play. *Nursing*, **4**(37), 8.

Stuart, G.W. and Sundeen, S.J. (1983) *Principles and Practice of Psychiatric Nursing*, 2nd edn, C.V. Mosby & Co, St Louis.

Turnquist, D.E., Harvey, J.H. and Anderson, B.C. (1988) Attributions and adjustment to life threatening illness. *British Journal of Clinical Psychology*, **27**, 55–65.

Webster, C. (1977) Nursing intervention in family abuse and violence, in *Principles of Psychiatric Nursing*, (eds G.W. Stuart and S.J. Sundeen), C.V. Mosby, St Louis, pp. 807–9.

World Health Organization (1977) *Alcohol Related Disability*, WHO, Geneva.

Yates, D.W., Hadfield, J.M. and Peters, S. (1987) Alcohol consumption of patients attending two accident and emergency departments in north west England. *Journal of the Royal Society of Medicine*, **80**, 486–9.

CHAPTER 3

Trauma centres in the UK: a nursing perspective

S. Davies and I. Wood

INTRODUCTION

One of the most popular debates in A and E nursing today continues to be centred around the provision of services for severely injured persons. This debate concerns all A and E nurses and must be extended into prehospital and rehabilitation as well as that care delivered in the A and E department. This chapter aims to explore some of the issues relating to trauma and arguments are centred around the concept of continuous trauma care within a wider trauma care network. To appreciate this concept the chapter considers how such a system may be organized in relation to a specific geographical area.

In addition, it is acknowledged that since the review of trauma services in the UK in the late 1980s, one of the arguments concerning A and E nurses has been related to the role of peripheral hospitals and trauma centres. Much of this debate has centred around potential changes to the role of the A and E nurse. This concern is addressed from a number of perspectives in this chapter and the points raised should be of interest to all nurses working in A and E.

This chapter, like all others in the book, relies upon the reader to pluck out relevant information and ideas and translate these into their own area of clinical practice via discussion with colleagues and users of the A and E service. Points for discussion should help the reader to examine information and arguments put forward.

The organization of the chapter into sections allows the reader to dip into parts of the chapter as required or alternatively it can be read from start to finish. As with other chapters within this book, it is anticipated that challenge of ideas will occur. This is welcomed and viewed as a means of broadening the debate surrounding trauma care within A and E nursing.

Finally, the reference list at the end of the chapter provides a rich source of supplementary reading for those who wish to take the subject further.

HISTORY OF TRAUMA SYSTEMS IN THE UK

The first example of a trauma care network in the UK can be traced back to the 1880s when Sir Robert Jones was appointed as the surgeon superintendent to the company constructing the Manchester Ship Canal (Seddon, 1961). During the six years of the construction many workers were injured and the death rate was particularly high. Recognizing this, Sir Robert took steps to develop a trauma care system. Along the length of the canal, a railway had been laid to supply the necessary materials for the canal's construction. Sir Robert made use of this facility to transport the injured workers to hospital. At either end of the railway, in Manchester and Liverpool, were hospitals designated to receive the injured men. At three positions along the canal there were hospitals staffed by a house surgeon and experienced nurses. If required, Sir Robert could be summoned by means of telegraph to the appropriate hospital. The train itself would blow a special whistle to prewarn the hospital staff of the arrival of an injured patient.

From this early example of a trauma care network, it can be seen that some of the ingredients necessary in the development of a trauma system were in place. These ingredients include an effective communication system and rapid transport facilities.

After this promising development, there was little progress in hospital trauma care in general. Once the patient arrived in hospital, much of the care was delivered by nurses and house surgeons (Drummond, 1980). It was not until experience was gained in dealing with battle casualties from world conflicts that some authorities saw the scope for improvement in the care of civilian trauma. To this end, in 1941 William Gissane was appointed director of the Queen's Hospital in Birmingham which was soon to become the Birmingham Accident Hospital (Harrison, 1984). In those early days, this facility combined many of the features seen today in a modern trauma centre such as resident consultant presence, communication between the ambulance and the admissions room and full surgical facilities (Drummond, 1980).

Over the next few decades, the Birmingham Accident Hospital gained a worldwide reputation in the treatment of trauma but despite its success the concept of an 'accident hospital' was not repeated

elsewhere in the UK. In the 1960s and early 1970s, various govern-
mental reports attempted to address the problems being experienced
in trauma care in the UK (Irving, 1989). It was not until 1971 that Bruce
recommended the establishment of 32 major Accident and Emergency
departments each under the direction of a consultant in Accident and
Emergency medicine. The value of A and E medicine was confirmed
by these reports and it is true to say that '. . . the specialty of Accident
and Emergency medicine has not looked back since that time' (Lewin,
1978).

OVERSEAS DEVELOPMENTS IN TRAUMA CARE

As with many historical innovations, the British lost their pioneering
lead to the North Americans. In 1965, there were some 107 000 killed
and over 10 000 000 people temporarily disabled as a result of accidental
injuries in the USA. These facts prompted the publication of a
document that could be seen as the foundation stone for the development of trauma care in the USA (National Academy of Sciences, 1966).
As a direct result of this work, trauma centres were gradually
developed in America. In 1976, the Committee on Trauma of the
American College of Surgeons began designating trauma centres as
levels I, II and III dependent on the facilities and resources available
and the total patient throughput in a year (Committee on Trauma of
the American College of Surgeons, 1990).

The level I centre has at its disposal emergency medicine and
anaesthesia together with all surgical specialities and these are available
24 hours a day on site. In addition to this, representatives from all
other medical specialities must be on call and promptly available. The
level I centre must also undertake teaching programmes for all staff
members in the institution. In addition, research projects looking into
trauma epidemiology, patient outcome and both nursing and medical
care strategies must be undertaken.

The level II centre has only to offer inhouse 24-hour a day emergency
medicine, general and neurosurgical facilities. Indeed, the initial
anaesthetic cover at such a facility may be offered by a certified
registered nurse anaesthetist (CRNA). This person is highly skilled
at advanced airway management, emergency induction of anaesthesia
and the performance of such procedures as central venous line
placement.

The level III centre is found in a more rural environment and only
has to provide an onsite emergency medicine capability. The
anaesthetic cover may again be provided by the CRNA with medical
anaesthetic back-up promptly available. General and neurosurgical
facilities need to be on call and promptly available.

In areas not served by a trauma centre, the mortality rate of road traffic accident victims was appreciably higher than in neighbouring areas that did possess a trauma centre facility. When the post mortem reports of road traffic accident victims were studied from two adjacent counties, two thirds of the non-central nervous system (CNS) related deaths and one third of CNS related deaths in the county with no trauma centre were judged to have been potentially preventable. Only one death in the county with a trauma centre was so judged (West *et al.*, 1979).

After the development of a trauma system, incorporating trauma centres, there was '... a severe reduction in the number of deaths judged preventable. In addition, a more aggressive approach to the traumatized patient was noted ...' (West *et al.*, 1983).

It would be a mistake to look upon the North American experience in isolation when considering the development of trauma care. Trunkey (1983) mentions that, 'One example of excellent regional trauma care can be found in West Germany'. In western Germany the system of trauma care entails a rapid prehospital land ambulance response. In addition, the use of helicopters based at 32 sites across the country facilitates the transport of the seriously injured to designated trauma centres. However, it may come as a surprise to UK nurses to realize that in Germany A and E departments simply do not exist as we know them. Likewise, the speciality of A and E medicine is not recognized.

Trauma centres in western Germany are staffed by a full surgical team with inhouse 24-hour consultant cover. In their system, the Germans were quick to seize on the need for an integral rehabilitation programme for the victims of trauma, '... the primary goal being to get the accident victim back to gainful employment as soon as possible' (Trunkey, 1983).

Within the trauma care network, some of the emergency response vehicles are staffed by doctors from the full range of specialities. On such vehicles, the doctor takes the lead with the paramedic taking a secondary role. Indeed, the paramedics can only perform such invasive tasks as endotracheal intubation under extreme circumstances, for example during a mass casualty situation. Such a response team may initially appear attractive when considering the management of seriously injured patients. However, one must remember that the doctor responding to such a patient may not have a trauma background and, indeed, they may be drawn from an unrelated speciality.

Points for discussion

● Given the difference in aetiology of trauma in the UK and the USA, is it correct to use the American model of trauma care when considering such developments in this country?

● Given that A and E departments in this country are staffed predominantly by junior medical staff, could there be a role for a nurse trained in the use of advanced airway management techniques similar to the American CRNA?

RECENT DEVELOPMENTS IN TRAUMA CARE IN THE UK

During the mid to late 1980s, increasing concern was again expressed in relation to the delivery of trauma care in the UK. Up to 20% of trauma deaths may well have been preventable; indeed, this figure may be as high as 33% (Anderson *et al.*, 1988). In 1988, the counterpart document to that produced in the USA some 22 years earlier was published by the Royal College of Surgeons of England. This report recommended that:

Patients with life threatening injury beyond the facilities and capabilities of the district general hospital should be transferred by high quality transport to a trauma centre established at regional or multidistrict level.

As a result of this report, the Department of Health agreed in 1990 to undertake an evaluation project into the feasibility of establishing trauma centres in the UK. Each regional health authority was asked to submit proposals for a pilot trauma centre in their region. A requirement for a hospital to be considered as a pilot centre was that it should serve a population of 2 million and offer the following facilities.

1. A and E and anaesthetic/ICU departments;
2. neurosurgery with onsite CT scanning;
3. all surgical specialities (cardiothoracic, ENT, faciomaxillary, general, ophthalmic, orthopaedic, plastic and urology).

Coincidentally during the late 1980s, steps were taken in establishing a trauma system in the north west Midlands (Templeton, 1991, personal communication). The focus of this system was an integrated approach to trauma care incorporating:

1. prehospital care – firm links were established with both the Staffordshire Ambulance Service and the Staffordshire Fire and Rescue Service;
2. hospital based care – a committee was formed, which meets on a regular basis to enable discussion between the surrounding hospitals in the North West Midlands Trauma System (NWMTS) (Fig. 3.1);

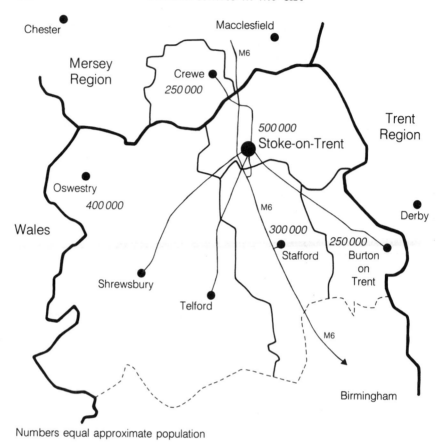

Numbers equal approximate population

Figure 3.1 North West Midlands trauma system.

3.   rehabilitation – the appointment of a consultant in rehabilitation medicine, together with the appointment of a brain injury research nurse.

Research within the NWMTS was undertaken to establish the nature, extent and severity of injuries encountered within the system (Maryosh *et al.*, 1991).

By the end of 1990, with this trauma system in its infancy, the North Staffordshire Hospital (NSH) in Stoke on Trent was chosen to be the pilot 'trauma centre' within the Department of Health Trauma Centre Evaluation Project (TCEP) (Redmond, 1992). The project provided funding for additional resources, including;

1.   three additional A and E consultants;
2.   two anaesthetic consultants with a main interest in trauma;

3. an increase in nursing establishment in A and E, operating department and intensive care;
4. an increase in radiography establishment;
5. provision of funding to enable A and E nurses to undertake provider courses in the Trauma Nurse Core Course (TNCC) (Emergency Nurses Association, 1988) and Advanced Trauma Nursing Course (ATNC) (American College of Surgeons, 1988);
6. purchase of a rapid infusion blood warmer and blood gas analyser for the A and E department.

An important feature of the developments at the NSH was the provision of 24-hour resident consultant cover to act as trauma team leaders in the A and E department. This was provided by the four A and E and the two anaesthetic consultants.

Two other hospitals, Royal Preston Hospital and Hull Royal Infirmary, were chosen to act as comparator sites for the TCEP. The Accident and Emergency departments at these hospitals were considered to be representative of facilities offering a good standard of trauma care. Additional funding made available to these departments would enable them to act as a baseline for comparison with the 'trauma centre' in Stoke.

A research team within the department of public health medicine at the University of Sheffield was established in order to undertake the scientific evaluation of the whole project.

Points for discussion

● How will the findings of the Sheffield research team shape the future of trauma care delivery in this country?

● Will the evaluation have to be repeated in other trauma systems in order to verify the data collected?

IMPLICATIONS FOR THE A AND E NURSE IN A TRAUMA CENTRE

Trauma training

Until recently, the training of nurses in relation to the assessment, management and care of trauma victims has largely been undertaken as part of the ENB 199 course in Accident and Emergency nursing. There has been great competition for places on such courses; however, the actual content relating to trauma management can vary significantly. As a result, it could be said that until recently trauma training for nurses in the UK had been fragmented and inconsistent.

This same inconsistency in training was also recognized within the medical profession. In an attempt to remedy this situation, some far-sighted individuals from both professions introduced recognized trauma training programmes from the USA. Nurses in the UK were introduced to the Trauma Nurse Core Course (TNCC) (ENA, 1988) and the Advanced Trauma Nursing Course (ATNC) whilst doctors took the direction of the Advanced Trauma Life Support Course (ATLS) (American College of Surgeons, 1993). These courses offer a standardized, systematic approach to the initial assessment, resuscitation and stabilization of the multiply injured patient.

Point for discussion

●   If all nurses and doctors working in A and E departments were to undertake one of the above courses, would it improve the outcome for the seriously injured patient?

Role expansion

The expanded role of the A and E nurse has largely been limited to the care of minor trauma victims with skills such as suturing, plastering and wound infiltration being the extent of practice in most A and E departments. Nurse involvement with the multiply injured patient offers a significant area for the development of interventional skills. The *Scope of Professional Practice* (UKCC, 1992) may open the way for nurses to undertake more interventionist role. This remains to be seen but it may remove much of the bureaucracy hitherto associated with expanded practice.

Points for discussion

●   Should all A and E nurses who care for seriously injured/ill patients be able to perform such skills as cannulation and endotracheal intubation?

●   How strenuously will nurses have to argue their case in order that they may undertake a more interventionist role?

Nurse's role in the trauma team

With the advent of standardized trauma training for the A and E nurse, their role in the trauma team can be considered from two aspects:

The senior nurse

This individual will have undertaken advanced trauma training and will, in conjunction with the medical trauma team leader, be responsible for the smooth running and organization of the trauma resuscitation. It is the responsibility of this nurse to ensure that nursing resources are allocated effectively within the trauma team. In liaison with the medical team leader, they will ensure that correct assessments and procedures are carried out in the correct order as established in the adopted protocol. Considerable preplanning and discussion at the departmental level involving all parties have to be undertaken to develop a standardized approach to trauma management.

The specific role of the senior trauma nurse would be agreed within individual departments but their responsibilities may include such areas as calculating the patient's trauma score, liaising with the X-ray department and arranging transport of blood specimens. In short, the role of the senior nurse is to conduct and coordinate the nursing section of the trauma team 'orchestra'.

The team nurse(s)

The role of the trauma team nurse will vary depending upon the prearranged and agreed departmental practice. Prior to the arrival of the patient, the senior nurse will allocate specific responsibilities to each nurse in turn according to laid down protocols. The individual team nurse(s) must ensure that they adhere to their allocated role unless directed otherwise by the senior trauma nurse. By doing this, they ensure that roles are not duplicated and effort not wasted.

The role of the team nurse offers scope for enhancement of practice. This may involve developing their clinical assessment skills such as chest auscultation, their practical skills such as cannulation and arterial blood gas sampling, and their interpersonal skills such as assertiveness.

There may be a school of thought within the nursing profession that believes that such interventions are not within the role of the nurse. If nurses do become more interventionist, they will need to develop greater proficiency in areas such as documentation skills so that effective audit can take place.

Points for discussion

● With the advent of increasing numbers of trained paramedics bringing trauma victims to A and E departments, would nurses have to stand aside whilst ambulance personnel perform life-saving skills which they themselves could be performing?

- If paramedic personnel are performing prehospital advanced life support interventions, do A and E nurses really need to be proficient in advanced skills?

- Would the nurse with expanded skills spend more time directly involved with their patient if they were performing interventions such as cannulation and venepuncture?

Departmental protocols

Staff allocation

Since the introduction of ATLS into this country in 1988, many A and E departments have revised their protocols for the assessment of trauma. With the need for rapid action within this framework, it may be necessary for nurses to have prearranged responsibilities in order to act speedily and effectively. The ATLS protocol focuses on the following headings and nurse's responsibilities within that protocol may be:

Airway with cervical spine control
Nurse 1 to work with doctor 1 to assess, manage and maintain a patent airway and to ensure cervical spine immobilization.

Breathing
Nurse 1 to work with doctor 1 to assess adequacy of respiratory effort, to intervene as appropriate and to maintain satisfactory ventilation.

Circulation
Nurse 2 to work with doctor 2 to assess circulatory effectiveness, to control haemorrhage and correct hypovolaemia. Maintain documentation in relation to the patient's physiological status.

Deficits
Nurse 2 to work with doctor 2 in assessing the patient's neurological function.

Exposure
Nurse 2 would expose the patient in readiness for the trauma team leader to direct a more detailed assessment of injury.

From the above protocol example, it can be seen that the role of each nurse is quite separate, thus ensuring no duplication of effort whilst at the same time ensuring that nothing that would compromise the patient's progress was omitted.

Points for discussion

● Is there scope for developing such a team approach within your A and E department?

● Are there the resources available to do so without compromising the care of the remaining patients?

Trauma protocols

Emergency departments may need to develop systems that rapidly identify the potentially seriously injured patient. From experience gained in the USA (West *et al.*, 1986) and under the direction of its consultants, the A and E department at the North Staffordshire Hospital has implemented a formal trauma protocol. The aim of the trauma protocol is to use the mechanism of a patient's injury as an indicator of the likelihood of significant trauma. Prior to its inception, patients were allocated to the resuscitation room largely as a result of a quick assessment by a trained nurse with their decision usually based on the appearance of any obvious presenting complaints.

Fig 3.2 shows the protocol for admission to the resuscitation area for all injured patients arriving with any of the listed criteria.

- Unconscious or significant history of unconsciousness
- Triage Revised Trauma Score less than 12
- Glasgow Coma Score less than 13
- Pedestrian struck by car
- Motorcyclist or cyclist (unless accident was low speed or stationary)
- Death of anyone in the accident
- Fall from a height greater than 15 feet
- Burns of 10% or more
- Inhalational burns
- Fractured shaft of femur
- More than one long bone fracture
- Possible cervical fracture
- More than one body compartment involved
- Patient ejected from vehicle
- Penetrating injury to head, chest or abdomen
- Entrapment for more than 20 minutes
- Amputation of a limb

Figure 3.2 North Staffordshire Hospital protocol for admission to resuscitation area.

The medical trauma leader is called by the senior nurse in the resuscitation room if the ambulance crew notify the A and E department to be on standby for the arrival of the patient.

The implementation of such protocols may lead to feelings of insecurity and role erosion amongst the nursing staff, who used to undertake the initial assessment of the newly arrived patient. Discussion should be undertaken between medical and nursing staff prior to the implementation of such a protocol so that professional concerns may be allayed.

Points for discussion

● How would you feel if, by implication, your decision making capabilities were questioned by medical staff?

● Could your department identify a greater number of seriously injured patients by using such a protocol?

● By allocating a trauma patient to a minor trauma area rather than to the resuscitation room, could it be said that staff in that area would label that patient as being a 'minor injury'? On the basis of being a 'minor injury', the patient may not receive a detailed examination when by the mechanism of his injury, he may indeed have a more serious underlying problem.

IMPLICATIONS FOR THE A AND E NURSE IN THE PERIPHERAL HOSPITAL

The concept of a multispeciality hospital at the hub of a trauma care system with several outlying hospital facilities serving it is a possible blueprint for the development of a comprehensive trauma service in the UK.

The extent to which the A and E nurse working in an outlying hospital would find their major trauma experience reduced may depend to a large extent upon the distances between their base hospital and the trauma centre. For example, in an area served by several hospitals sited only a few miles part, the journey time from the accident scene may justify the nearest hospital being bypassed and the patient being taken to the most appropriate hospital; that is, the trauma centre. Conversely, in an area in which the peripheral hospitals are remote and the journey times much greater, the potential for direct admission to the trauma centre may not be as great. In this situation, the nurse at the peripheral hospital will need to acquire more advanced skills as they would be required to escort the now stabilized trauma patient on their journey to the trauma centre. The interhospital transfer of patients may well be an area in which these nurses can develop a particular expertise.

One way in which nurses from the periphery may be better integrated into the trauma system would be for the development of a facility for such nurses to enter an exchange programme with their colleagues working in the trauma centre. In this way, they would continue to develop their experience in dealing with the multiply injured patient, gain exposure to the working atmosphere within the trauma centre and gather ideas to take back to their base hospital. The trauma centre nurses exchanged to the peripheral hospital may well be able to impart some of their expertise. However, the manner in which this is done must be sensitive to the feelings of the local A and E staff.

Both of the above strategies may contribute to the development of a feeling of esprit de corps within the trauma system and thus ensure that the multiply injured patient and their family receives the best possible care.

Points for discussion

● How does the nurse working within the peripheral hospital feel when a large proportion of seriously injured patients either bypass their hospital or are admitted for assessment and are rapidly transferred out to the trauma centre?

● How can the nurses in the peripheral hospitals, who may find their exposure to major trauma reduced when their departments are bypassed, develop their trauma related skills?

TRANSPORT WITHIN A TRAUMA SYSTEM

Adams Cowley in Baltimore clearly demonstrated the importance of getting the trauma victim quickly from the incident scene to definitive care (Cowley *et al.*, 1973). In order to facilitate this rapid intervention, the system will need to develop an efficient and effective transport network. Integral in this development will be the ambulance service. In developing a trauma system it is important that close links are established at an early stage with the ambulance services involved. The senior ambulance officers should be present at all important planning meetings in order that full consultation can include the extent and nature of any developments necessary within the trauma system. Such developments may include an increased number of paramedics undergoing training and the integration of rapid response paramedic vehicles into the existing ambulance network. Such an increase in paramedic training programmes may have an effect on nurses working in A and E in that they may be asked to take on the role of facilitator/educator for the trainees during their allocation to the A and E department.

If trauma centres are to be established in the UK, such centres must serve a large enough geographical area to ensure that sufficient patient throughput is maintained. Only by exposing both the staff and the system to sufficient volume of trauma patients will the necessary skills and expertise be achieved and maintained.

As discussed earlier, the travelling times for trauma victims in large conurbations may be sufficiently short for satisfactory land ambulance transfer direct to the trauma centre. If, however, the transfer time from the periphery of the system is prolonged or if road traffic congestion leads to delays, there may be a need for an alternative mode of transport. Until relatively recently, the UK has been slow to seize upon the idea of using civilian helicopters in medical scenarios. The lead in this area was taken by the Cornwall Ambulance Service in 1987 when they established an air ambulance service. Since then there has been sporadic introduction of further air ambulances (Delamothe, 1989). Many of these are under the direct control of the relevant ambulance services. However, some are primarily police helicopters with an ambulance paramedic on board so that the facility can be sent to accidents as required.

To date, only one medical response helicopter is hospital based, at the rooftop helipad of the Royal London Hospital in Whitechapel. It is known as the HEMS (Helicopter Emergency Medical Service) (Earlam and Wilson, 1989). This helicopter provides a service primarily for the area within the M25 motorway surrounding the capital. With London's inherent traffic congestion, the speed with which the HEMS can respond to incidents and transport the injured victim to the appropriate facility may well be a definite improvement on the existing land ambulance service. In measuring the success of such a rapid intervention system, due consideration must be given to the fact that the HEMS helicopter is the only one in the UK which carries a paramedic **and** a doctor at all times.

The role of helicopters in emergency medical services in the UK is at present being evaluated by the department of public health medicine at the University of Sheffield.

The use of helicopters in emergency care has several limitations. They are undeniably expensive to operate and maintain; they cannot fly in adverse weather conditions or at night unless specially equipped; access to the patient is restricted in certain types of helicopter and it may be difficult to transport certain categories of patient due to the particular design of the helicopter. In particular, it may be inappropriate to transport the pregnant patient or the person with a mental health problem by helicopter. It is desirable that the helicopter lands on a designated landing site adjacent to the trauma centre. Few large hospitals in the UK currently possess such ideal facilities and, as a consequence, the final leg of the journey from landing site to A and E is made by land ambulance. This negates some of the benefits in reduced transport time made by the helicopter.

There is evidence to suggest that the time of helicopter deployment to the incident is crucial if transport time savings are to be maximized (Rouse, 1992). In order to facilitate such savings, it may be beneficial to have a helicopter paramedic allocated to the ambulance control in order to triage the '999 emergency' calls and to send the helicopter at the appropriate time to the appropriate incident. In doing this, the helicopter would possibly respond to an incident without waiting to be called by a land ambulance crew.

Helicopters are ideally suited to the task of secondary transfer of patients to the trauma centre from a peripheral hospital. It is in the area of interhospital transfer that there would appear to be scope for nurses to develop expertise.

Points for discussion

- Is there a role for the A and E nurse as part of the prehospital care team?
- Could a nurse be of value on a helicopter or as a third crew member alongside a paramedic and a technician on an emergency ambulance?
- Do you know how to approach a helicopter that is about to land next to your department?
- Would you know how to assist in the unloading of the patient from the helicopter?
- Should a nurse have an input into the planning of a trauma system transport network?

COMMUNICATIONS WITHIN A TRAUMA SYSTEM

Parallel to the development of the transport network within the trauma system must be the enhancement of the communications facility. This will primarily be the remit of the ambulance services. Many A and E departments now have a radio link with the ambulance controls serving the department. It is possible to have direct 'talk through' from the A and E department to the vehicles whilst they are en route to the hospital. This facility allows for detailed information to be available to the staff in the receiving department prior to the patient's arrival. It is important that A and E nurses using such a 'talk through' facility are both confident and fully conversant with the use of radio procedure. A and E nurse managers should ensure that by liaising with the ambulance communications manager, they provide a teaching programme for the A and E nurse to become more proficient in the use of the radio facility.

Having delivered the patient to A and E, it is essential that the ambulance crew provide a written record detailing patient information and emergency interventions carried out in the prehospital phase. Such standardized patient report forms have been developed in an attempt to formalize a tool for prehospital care audit (Nichol, 1991). In the current Department of Health Trauma Centre Evaluation Project, identical prehospital patient report forms have been developed and are being evaluated in each of the participating areas. Nurses may have a role in the future evolution of such data collection as it is they who have to interpret such reports upon the patient's arrival in A and E and transpose such information into the individual's A and E notes.

Recent developments in telecommunications such as cellular telephones may have a role within the trauma system communications network. Perhaps by providing each ambulance paramedic and each consultant at adjacent A and E departments with a cellular telephone or a handheld radio, personal communication with the trauma team leader at the trauma centre may be enhanced. In such a system, a conversation involving all three parties could be used as a mechanism for deciding the most appropriate receiving facility for a given trauma victim.

In the near future, the use of information technology may allow for the seamless passage of detailed patient data from the prehospital arena to the A and E department and beyond.

Point for discussion

● Should there be a nurse representative involved in the development of enhanced communications systems?

NURSING MANAGEMENT IN THE TRAUMA CENTRE

In an earlier section we suggested that nurses working in a trauma centre may develop feelings of insecurity and role conflict regarding their position within the system. It is important to remember that it is often the nursing team that coordinates and manages an A and E department on a daily basis and as such the need for strong and effective nursing leadership is important.

In developing a trauma centre, nursing involvement in the planning procedure must be undertaken from the beginning. Consideration needs to be given to the formation of a nursing strategy. Such a strategy will include recruitment and retention of staff, stress management issues, postregistration education needs, budgetary/resource considerations, staffing levels and interprofessional issues (Beachley and Snow, 1988).

In the following section, we aim to discuss the above nursing strategy components and offer some ideas for consideration.

Recruitment and retention of staff

It could be suggested that nurses working in A and E departments have chosen this career pathway because they relish the unpredictability and excitement of working in an area that offers many different challenges and experiences. It is known that nurses derive greatest satisfaction from caring for 'good' patient events such as cardiac arrests and major trauma (Jeffery, 1979). In order to fulfil these needs, many nurses wish to work in a department that offers them an increased exposure to the types of experiences that make the job interesting, so that recruitment and retention of staff may not be perceived as a problem when developing an overall nursing strategy for a trauma centre. However, unless clear career development possibilities are available within the trauma centre and/or the professional development of nursing staff is both encouraged and facilitated, experienced and valued staff may not be retained. By adequate forward planning, the retention of staff can be considered when the nurse is first interviewed for employment. By defining at interview the areas in which each individual nurse wishes their career to develop, a manager will have the opportunity to decide which nurse is suitable for employment and whether that individual's career needs can be accommodated within the existing organization.

Points for discussion

● How much consideration is given to recruitment and retention in your present A and E nursing strategy?

● How much scope is there for developing a recruitment strategy within your present organization?

Stress management

Without doubt, the stresses experienced by staff working in a trauma centre with a high throughput of seriously injured patients will be accentuated. When considering the effects such stressors will have on individuals, one must also be mindful of the cumulative effect of any additional developments that have been implemented. These may include the introduction of trauma protocols, orientation of additional nursing and medical staff, familiarization with new equipment and the space available to accommodate the extra patient throughput. At present formalized stress management facilities are available for use by multidisciplinary staff groups (National Health Service Training Authority, 1990). Within the trauma situation, it has been suggested that time must be made available for a postresuscitation debrief in order that the trauma team, including the ambulance personnel involved, can attend to any issues that cause them concern. In such debrief situations, it is important that due consideration is given to the feelings and concerns of individual members of the team and that any shortcomings identified are dealt with sensitively.

Point for discussion

● With the demands placed on existing resources, would time be made available for staff to debrief after a trauma resuscitation?

Postregistration training needs

One of the most important aspects to consider when developing a trauma system is the enhanced training required by both nurses and doctors working in the A and E department. In recent years, great improvements have been made in the quality and availability of both adult and paediatric advanced trauma nursing courses. Such courses are designed to enable nurses working within a trauma team to assess and manage a given patient along the same protocols as the doctors dealing with the patient.

In addition to trauma nursing courses, consideration should be given to the need to develop cardiac life support, airway management, cannulation, defibrillation and counselling skills to deal with distressed relatives. If nurses are to become involved in rapid response teams from the A and E department, they will need to undertake specialist training relating to patient management in the prehospital environment. Such courses are being developed at present.

Undoubtedly, in the world of emergency medical services there will be an increasing use of computers and information technology in general. As a consequence of this there will be a need for nurses to become more conversant with their use.

Budgetary/resource considerations

Newly instituted treatment protocols may require the purchase of more varied consumable items such as non re-breathing oxygen masks, rigid cervical spine immobilization devices and pressure transducer sets. In addition to these consumable items, the trauma centre may need to invest in more expensive therapeutic/diagnostic equipment such as rapid infusion blood warming capability and blood gas analysis equipment. All these developments place demands on what may be an already stretched budget.

Staffing levels

As a consequence of increased trauma patient throughput, it would seem obvious that an increase in nursing establishment would be required if management of such traumatized patients is to be carried out effectively. Such an increase will have budgetary considerations similar to those mentioned above. When addressing the issue of staffing levels, it is important to realize that the care delivered to the other A and E patients may be adversely affected if there is no increase in establishment. Given that the A and E nurse will have to respond rapidly to the arrival of a greater number of major trauma patients, it can be seen that the attention accorded to the less seriously ill/injured will be reduced. It is important that the senior nurse on duty gives due consideration to the needs of the less seriously ill/injured and allocates nursing resources accordingly.

Interprofessional issues

Within the trauma centre, the trauma team is truly multidisciplinary. The dynamics of such an organization are complex and in managing a team which has to function and work so closely together, some mechanism for dialogue between the team members has to be instituted. This dialogue may take place at regular meetings between the parties involved in which new ideas and problems can be discussed in a frank and forthright manner.

RESEARCH AND DATA COLLECTION

The management of the traumatized patient has provided the basis for much valuable medical and nursing research and continues to do so. In auditing the outcome of trauma victims it is important that all emergency care facilities use the same research methodology so that one is comparing like with like. At present in the UK the trauma audit tool in use is the TRISS (Trauma Score and Injury Severity Score) (Boyd *et al.*, 1987). At first this may seem quite complex to the A and E nurse but it is essential that they have a basic understanding of trauma scoring so that they realize the importance of gathering the correct physiological data (Davies *et al.*, 1992). Evaluation of the management and the final outcome of the trauma patient must be undertaken in order to establish the effectiveness of the care delivery within the trauma system. Inclusion of a given trauma centre/A and E department within the UK Major Trauma Outcome Study (Yates *et al.*, 1992) will allow departmental performance to be measured so that areas that require improvement may be identified.

The extent of UK nursing research into trauma management has been limited to date when compared with the level of work conducted in the USA. However, in recent years more and more A and E nurses have become aware of the value of research in the clinical area. In the implementation of a trauma centre many avenues for research may be opened up, thus allowing for an atmosphere conducive to both nursing and multidisciplinary research. It may well be appropriate to appoint a nurse from within the department to include research as part of their job description. Such an individual, whilst having a challenging and rewarding experience, would have to work closely with their A and E colleagues in order to generate a clinical climate conducive to accurate data collection.

REHABILITATION AS A COMPONENT OF A TRAUMA SYSTEM

The element of a trauma care network that is most commonly forgotten is rehabilitation. The individual nurse working in a rehabilitative setting may well have different beliefs, values and expectations of the trauma patient from their colleague working in Accident and Emergency. Whilst often overlooked by nurses working in A and E, it is valuable to realize that the rehabilitation of the trauma victim should start at the point of entry into the hospital.

With experience gained in major trauma management and improved treatment protocols, some patients will survive who hitherto may well have died. These patients might well be left with a degree of physical and/or mental disability following their injury and it is important that the quality of life experienced by these individuals is maximized. By considering such issues as care of pressure areas and positioning of limbs, nurses working in A and E can play their part in the rehabilitation process. In addition to the patient, due consideration must be given to the needs of relatives and loved ones with respect to the patient's possible future disabilities and how this may affect them.

It is important that any goals set in the rehabilitative phase are realistically attainable; if they are not, conflict may well ensue.

FUTURE DEVELOPMENTS

In the early 1990s, government policy encouraged the establishment of NHS trusts. This policy is an attempt to devolve organizational responsibility for health care to a more local level. With the advent of such trusts has come the concept of purchasers and providers of health care services. Trauma centres, if established in the UK, would be providers of health care with the trauma facility having its services purchased either by local health authorities or other NHS hospital trusts.

Such a situation can be considered in two ways. Firstly, by undertaking a large major trauma patient throughput, the trauma centre will develop experience and expertise in the management of such cases. By so doing, early definitive management should lead to a better quality of care and, hence, the patient's length of stay in hospital can be reduced. By reducing inpatient hospital costs, particularly in intensive care, the trauma centre may offer better value for money for the purchasing authority.

However, the prevalence of severe head injuries in major trauma cases may mean that a percentage of patients referred to the trauma centre require prolonged intensive care and rehabilitation. Unfortunately, the care of such individuals will inevitably be more expensive. When negotiating referral contracts, the trauma centre providing the services must be careful to take account of the approximate numbers of such patients that it is likely to receive in a given financial year. Failure to do so may have severe resource implications for the centre.

Within any trauma system there may be a need to establish a coordinator role between the various agencies involved. This role in the United States has been undertaken by a trauma nurse coordinator (Beachley *et al.*, 1988). In the UK the role of this coordinator may involve work in developing the system at a regional level. Conversely, the coordinator may have a role in developing the integrated approach of all components of the hospital response. By the examples given it can be seen that there may be a role for two such nurse coordinators within any given trauma system. Certainly, quality assurance and audit would be of importance within the remit of any coordinating nurse.

The current gap between the A and E department and the ambulance service will have to be reduced if a truly integrated approach to trauma care is to be established in the UK. By integrating the services, the ambulance crews could gather experience within the hospital environment whilst remaining available for immediate response to emergency calls.

Points for discussion

● Can it be speculated that rather than provide the full range of services necessary for the care of severely injured patients, a given NHS hospital trust may wish to refer more of their severely injured patients to a trauma centre and, by so doing, make more effective use of financial resources?

● Would it be attractive for the referring hospital to transfer to the trauma centre its potentially complex trauma patients whose continuing rehabilitative care may otherwise involve heavy financial costs to the initial receiving hospital?

● Will the provision of trauma services in the future be determined by business managers with budgets rather than by clinicians?

● Would it be feasible for paramedic ambulance personnel to have their vehicles based outside the trauma centre?

● Should the need arise, could a doctor or nurse from the trauma centre be called upon to respond with the ambulance crew to the emergency (Angell Garza, 1990)?

The Department of Health Trauma Centre Evaluation Project currently being undertaken in the north west Midlands is designed to appraise the appropriateness of establishing trauma centres across the UK. If this project proves that trauma centres do provide a better outcome for the victims of trauma, it may be that 20–25 such systems would evolve around a corresponding trauma centre. The sites for such trauma systems would be decided by geographic population served and the trauma centre by the facilities available on site.

Point for discussion

● Will this mean that trauma systems are focused around university teaching hospitals which already have many of the key ingredients in place necessary for the formation of a trauma centre?

The role of the trauma nurse is yet to evolve fully in the UK. There are those who believe that nurses should nurse and there are those who believe that the nurse should become more interventionist. Whoever is right, the role of the trauma nurse will change if the establishment of trauma centres becomes a reality in this country. For those nurses who wish to become more interventionist, there will almost certainly be an increased scope within such centres for them to develop both personally and professionally.

REFERENCES

American College of Surgeons Committee on Trauma (1990) Resources for Optimal Care of the Injured Patient, American College of Surgeons, Chicago.

American College of Surgeons Committee on Trauma (1993) Advanced Trauma Life Support Course, American College of Surgeons, Chicago.

Anderson, I.D., Woodford, M., De Dombal, T. and Irving, M. (1988) Retrospective study of 1000 deaths from injury in England and Wales. *British Medical Journal*, **296**, 1305–8.

Angell Garza, M. (1990) Trading places – paramedics in the hospitals, nurses in the field. *Journal of Emergency Medical Services*, **15**(2), 56–65.

Beachley, M. and Snow, S. (1988) Developing trauma care systems: a nursing perspective. *Journal of Nursing Administration*, **18**(4), 22–9.

Beachley, M., Snow, S. and Trimble, P. (1988) Developing trauma care systems: the trauma nurse coordinator. *Journal of Nursing Administration*, **18**(7), 34–42.

Boyd, C.R., Tolson, M.A. and Copes, W.S. (1987) Evaluating trauma care: the TRISS method. *Journal of Trauma*, **27**(4), 370–8.

Bruce, J. (1971) *Report of the Joint Working Party*, Joint Consultants Committee, British Medical Association, London.

Cowley, R.A., Hudson, F., Scanlan, E. *et al.* (1973) An economical and proved helicopter programme for transporting emergency critically ill and injured patients in Maryland. *Journal of Trauma*, **13**, 1029.

Davies, S., Hill, P., Wood, I.M. and Maryosh, J. (1992) Assessing trauma. *Nursing Times*, **88**(17), 54–7.

Delamothe, T. (1989) Here come the helicopters. *British Medical Journal*, **299**, 639.

Drummond, P. (1980) Trauma – the way to cope? *Health and Social Services Journal*, **90**, 1126–30.

Earlam, R. and Wilson, A. (1989) Helicopter Emergency Medical Services – HEMS One. *Annals of the Royal College of Surgeons of England*, **71**(4), 60–4.

Emergency Nurses Association (1988) Trauma Nurse Core Course (Provider), 2nd edn, Emergency Nurses Association, Chicago.

Harrison, S.H. (1984) Accident surgery – the life and times of William Gissane. *Injury*, **16**(3), 145–54.

Irving, M. (1989) The evolution of trauma care in the United Kingdom. *Injury*, **20**(6), 317–21.

Jeffery, R. (1979) Normal rubbish: deviant patients in casualty departments. *Sociology of Health and Illness*, **1**(1), 90–107.

Lewin, W. (1978) *Medical Staffing of Accident and Emergency Departments*, Joint Consultants Committee, British Medical Association, London.

Maryosh, J., Johnstone, S., Templeton, J. *et al.* (1991) *An Incidence Study of Trauma in the North Staffordshire Health District*, Department of Orthopaedic Surgery, Keele University.

National Academy of Sciences/National Research Council (1966) *Accidental Death and Disability: The Neglected Disease of Modern Society*, 1071–A–13, Committee on Trauma and Committee on Shock, Division of Medical Sciences, Washington DC.

National Health Service Training Authority (1990) *Health Pick-up. 'Managing Your Stress'*, NHSTA, London.

Nichol, J. (1991) Personal communication.

Redmond, A.D. (1992) UK trauma centres. *Hospital Update*, **18**, 699–705.

Rouse, A. (1992) The effect of the Cornwall and Isles of Scilly helicopter ambulance unit on the ambulance services' ability to deliver acutely traumatised patients to hospital. *Archives of Emergency Medicine*, **9**, 113–21.

Royal College of Surgeons of England/Commission on the Provision of Surgical Services (1988) *Report of the Working Party on the Management of Patients with Major Injuries*, RCS, London.

Seddon, H.J. (1961) The Manchester Ship Canal and the colonial frontier. *Journal of Bone and Joint Surgery*, **43**B(3), 425–9.

Trunkey, D.D. (1983) Trauma. *Scientific American*, **249**(2), 20–7.

United Kingdom Central Council (1992) *The Scope of Professional Practice*, UKCC, London.

West, J.G., Cales, R.H. and Gazzaniga, A.B. (1983) Impact of regionalization. The Orange County experience. *Archives of Surgery*, **118**, 740–4.

West, J.G., Murdock, M.A., Baldwin, L.C. and Whalen, K. (1986) A method for evaluating field triage criteria. *Journal of Trauma*, **26**(7), 655–9.

West, J.G., Trunkey, D.D. and Lim, R.C. (1979) Systems of trauma care. A study of two counties. *Archives of Surgery*, **114**, 455–9.

Yates, D.W., Woodford, M. and Hollis, S. (1992) Preliminary analysis of the care of injured patients in 33 British hospitals: first report of the United Kingdom major trauma outcome study. *British Medical Journal*, **305**, 737–40.

CHAPTER 4

The development of trauma education for A and E nurses in the UK

L. Hadfield-Law

INTRODUCTION

Trauma is a health problem and A and E nurses need to be prepared to deal with the many aspects of trauma competently and confidently. The introduction of a number of trauma care initiatives has raised awareness of the role of the A and E nurse in the resuscitation room. In particular the role of the nurse as coordinator of care is now being addressed. Such a role requires examination of confidence: confidence to communicate with as well as the ability to contribute to the multidisciplinary team within the resuscitation room.

This chapter will raise a number of questions as well as provide a wealth of information relating to the preparation of nurses in relation to care of the person following trauma. The chapter concentrates upon care of the adult in the A and E resuscitation room although it is acknowledged that children may be victims of trauma and that care of the person following trauma may begin in the prehospital setting and continue far beyond the A and E department.

Inherent within the chapter is the confidence versus competence debate and readers may wish to consider whether time spent working in A and E prepares nurses sufficiently to coordinate care for the multiply injured person and the person following trauma. Points for discussion are used to help the reader explore various aspects of the chapter and readers are expected to analyse their own position in relation to their own knowledge and skill and how both may be demonstrated in the resuscitation room.

Information relating to the content of two trauma training courses is presented within the chapter and readers are invited to consider such information within their own departments and in relation to their own experiences of caring for patients following trauma. As a result of this some readers may feel uncomfortable about their own competence. If this occurs, it is considered a positive outcome of the chapter as it is believed that such concern will lead to further examination of personal knowledge, skill and performance in the resuscitation room. For those nurses wishing to know more about such courses, information is available at the end of the chapter. In addition the references at the end of the chapter provide a basis for extra reading and should be followed up by the reader as necessary.

MAJOR TRAUMA

Major trauma can result in death within seconds; survivors have multiple injuries and are vulnerable to imminent death during the subsequent couple of hours. This critical time period is known as the 'golden hour' (Cowley, 1976).

Major trauma is the killer of one of our country's most valuable resources – young people. It is the commonest cause of death in the under-35 age group. Members of this group have families, dependants and jobs. In Britain, 22 000 lives are lost each year as the result of trauma (WHO, 1989). Road traffic accidents kill around 100 individuals a week (OPCS, 1991).

This handful of British statistics illustrates the tremendous health problem facing our country. Few can afford multiple injuries and their aftermath, not just in financial terms but in terms of pain and human suffering. There is no evidence to suggest that this problem is a new one but it has taken some time for those concerned with health care and politics to recognize its magnitude. The NHS Management Executive (DoH, 1992) have identified accidents as one of the five key areas where health care professionals will need to focus improvements for 1992–1994.

Point for discussion

● What methods may be used to raise public awareness of the magnitude of trauma as a health care problem?

In 1988, the Royal College of Surgeons of England published a report on the care of patients with major injuries in England and Wales. Evidence suggested that at least 2700 multiply injured patients die unnecessarily each year. Yates *et al.* (1992) concluded that the initial management of major trauma remains unsatisfactory. Mortality varies inexplicably between hospitals. Death is not, of course, the only negative performance indicator. It is suggested that for every trauma death, two more individuals are rendered permanently disabled (American College of Surgeons, 1989).

Points for discussion

● What kinds of physical and psychosocial problems will face individuals rendered permanently disabled due to trauma?

● What areas of accident prevention might be appropriately explored by nurses?

These unnecessary deaths and disabilities are not the result of complicated conditions, which are difficult to recognize, but often are due to hypoxia, hypovolaemia, missed diagnosis or delayed operation (Anderson, *et al.* 1988). Having begun to assess the extent of the problem, it is now time to address solutions as a nation. Clearly the best solution is accident prevention, responsibility for which lies with many individuals and organizations. Once a trauma patient has sustained injuries and has passed through the prehospital care phase, Accident and Emergency staff are responsible for receiving them at the hospital. Staff may be organized into a formal trauma team which functions in a similar way to a resuscitation team or, as is the more usual case, several nurses, doctors, porters, radiographers and other personnel are present, with no specific or predesignated roles.

Points for discussion

● Identify those individuals who may assume roles within the trauma team.

● What benefits maybe derived from joint training programmes?

To perform well, teams require organization and training, a co-ordinated approach subscribed to and understood by all members and mutual trust and respect amongst those team members. It is said that one of the best ways to develop mutual trust and respect is to participate in joint training programmes (Myers and Hopperstead, 1982). Learning seems to be enhanced by shared experiences. This chapter will focus on training opportunities for the nurse as part of the trauma team in Britain. The ATNC course will be identified, its content outlined and its accessibility discussed (Hadfield, 1993).

Points for discussion

● What benefits may be derived from joint training programmes?

● What difficulties might face those developing joint training programmes?

● Do you consider that excellent standards pertaining to the care of the trauma patient depend on experience or training?

THE ROLE OF THE TRAUMA NURSE

Effective care of the multiply injured patient relies very heavily on a consistent, coordinated approach with an organized system of care (Trauma Nursing Coalition, 1992). It has been suggested that the most significant ingredient for excellent care of the trauma patient is commitment. Recent steps forward in terms of resuscitation, diagnostic testing and new technology should not be underestimated but the role of each individual trauma team member is of key importance. Nurses are able to make a unique contribution to the care of the multiply injured patient. Nevertheless the role of the trauma nurse interfaces with those of other members within the trauma team, which may consist of an informal group of individuals who care for the multiply injured patient or a more formal resuscitation team identified as 'the trauma team'.

The nursing contribution to optimal trauma care during the 'golden hour' (Cowley, 1976) can be divided into seven areas:

1. assessment and intervention;
2. communication;
3. evaluation;
4. documentation;
5. planning;
6. debriefing;
7. advocacy.

(Hadfield, 1992)

Assessment

Assessment is the vital initial step in the care of the trauma patient. The nurse is usually the first member of the trauma team to receive the multiply injured patient into the A and E department. She will often remain with the patient throughout his stay in A and E and his transfer to definitive care. In view of this, the trauma nurse must be able to perform a rapid and effective initial assessment of the patient. To complete a comprehensive assessment, the nurse must be able to recognize:

● airway obstruction;
● potential for cervical spine injury;
● the need to call for assistance;

- breathing difficulties;
- possible chest injury;
- hypovolaemic, cardiogenic and neurogenic shock;
- how much intravascular volume has been lost and from where;
- neurological injury;
- the need for staff and patient protection from infection.

In addition the nurse must be able to prevent the deterioration of the trauma patient due to:

- airway obstruction;
- spinal cord injury;
- inadequate ventilation;
- circulatory collapse;
- secondary brain injury.

Augmenting an adequate knowledge base to recognize life and limb-threatening problems, and to prevent further harm to the patient, various psychomotor skills are required to provide safe and efficient care. Nursing responsibilities towards injured patients include the performance of life-saving manoeuvres; the following must be competently and quickly performed by any nurse receiving the trauma patient.

Airway control

- suction techniques;
- chin lift and jaw thrust manoeuvres;
- insertion of oro/nasopharyngeal airways;
- anticipation of equipment required for needle/surgical cricothyroidotomy and urgent oro/nasal intubation.

Cervical spine protection

- manual immobilization of the cervical spine;
- correct sizing of rigid cervical collar;
- safe application and removal of the cervical collar;
- immobilization of the patient's cervical spine in addition to collar application.

Assistance with breathing

- administration of high flow oxygen;
- positive pressure ventilation with bag-valve mask technique;
- anticipate equipment required for needle cricothyroidotomy and chest drain insertion;
- correct covering of open pneumothorax.

Control of circulatory loss

- application of external pressure to bleeding points;
- assistance in replacing intravascular fluid loss.

Maintenance of spinal immobilization

- safe and effective log rolling;
- straight lifting of the patient with potential spinal injury.

Accurate assessment of the trauma patient should happen swiftly and in conjunction with an appropriate resuscitation. Actual and potential injuries must be identified. Baselines and subsequent response to interventions should be recorded.

Initial assessment of the trauma patient follows the ATNC/TNCC format. During the primary survey, life-threatening injuries are identified and resuscitation initiated. Assessment strictly adheres to the system of:

A – Airway with cervical spine immobilization
B – Breathing
C – Circulation with haemorrhage control
D – Disability; assessment of neurological status
E – Exposure

The resuscitation phase runs concurrently with the primary survey. By rigidly adhering to such a system, no actual or potential life-threatening injury is missed by the team, thus achieving optimal patient outcome.

Communication

Communication is a process by which a message acts as a linkage between people (Glasser, 1989). Effective communication is an important component of cohesive team effort. A communication network with the patient as the central focus will support the system required to ensure good patient outcome. The trauma nurse, by fulfilling her role as communicator and advocate, is the most important link between the patient and the trauma team (Carl and Champion, 1986). If the communication network breaks down, the outcome can be disastrous.

During resuscitation the trauma nurse is responsible for supervising nursing activities within the trauma team, and for communicating with other team members.

The nurses are also an important link between the patient and their loved ones. Trauma catches family and friends completely unprepared; they have had no time to build up a protective shell. These people are at special risk and their needs require special attention.

Not only does effective communication ensure safe and timely patient care, it is also the single most important legal responsibility of the nurse. The nurse may be liable for failure to communicate at the right time, in the right way, to the right person.

Points for discussion

● What factors may contribute to the breakdown in the communication network surrounding the trauma patient?

● Identify the aspects of trauma patient care which require careful documentation.

Evaluation

A nurse would usually remain with the patient throughout his stay in the A and E department up to definitive care. This puts her in a unique position to pick up subtle changes in the patient's condition. The nurse has a primary responsibility to evaluate the patient's responses to therapeutic interventions by collecting data which reflect the response to and extent of injury. To be alert to subtle changes in condition, the nurse must be aware of acceptable parameters. It is essential that the nurse understands the physiological response to shock and the signs and symptoms associated with this. It is also important that the nurse has the required skills to take all the patient's vital signs including:

- temperature;
- pulse;
- respirations;
- blood pressure;
- capillary refill;
- neurological assessment.

It is important that she is not only able to pick up subtle changes in the patient's condition but that she understands what these might mean and is aware of who to pass the information on to.

Trauma scoring can be used by nurses to assess the level of care required by individual patients. The Revised Trauma Score is a numerical value derived from the respiratory, cardiovascular and central nervous system responses to injury. From this score, an estimate can be made regarding how severe the patient's injuries are (Davies, 1993). Such information can also be very valuable when considering audit of patient care.

Documentation

Documentation of assessment and intervention data can be a time consuming problem in a situation where little time exists. However, the patient notes provide a record of clinical care, data for audit and research and evidence in the event of medico-legal review. They provide a chronological record of patient treatment, patient's response to treatment and the means to review the quality of care (Trauma Nursing Coalition, 1992). Fully comprehensive documentation is one of the most important risk reduction strategies for the trauma team. During resuscitation the patient's condition can change dramatically and very rapidly and documentation of assessment, intervention, response and timing is essential to prove optimal patient care delivery.

To provide comprehensive and accurate documentation, it is important for the recorder to have sound clinical knowledge. The trauma nurse is very well placed to assume this role. This nurse should remain with the patient throughout resuscitation to definitive care and should document all data required. The trauma nurse should act as the central focus for all written and verbal communication during the resuscitation.

The use of trauma resuscitation flow sheets can save a great deal of time, ensure structured records and act as an aide-memoire.

Point for discussion

● Identify the aspects of trauma patient care which require careful documentation.

Planning

Planning ahead is an essential component of trauma nursing. Planning for the receipt of the trauma patient involves the creation of a suitable trauma room environment. Health and safety issues affecting the resuscitation area need to be considered. Appropriate environmental design of the resuscitation room is also important if the trauma team is to function effectively. Methods of orientating new staff to the resuscitation room need to be developed. Appropriate equipment needs to be prepared for the admission of the trauma patient, as well as the safe transfer of the patient to other areas.

Patients must be protected from wound contamination and both staff and patients from the transmission of bloodborne diseases. All trauma nurses must be aware of the recommended procedures for the prevention of transmission of human immunodeficiency virus (HIV) or hepatitis (Halpern, 1987).

Once trauma resuscitation is in progress the trauma nurse must always be one step ahead of the rest of the team. She will need to consider where the patient will be in ten minutes time. By doing this, valuable minutes can be saved by anticipating what the patient will need and where he will be going.

Point for discussion

● What preparation will the trauma nurse need to make prior to the arrival of the patient?

Debriefing

Exposure to high levels of stress has been identified as one of the main reasons for the high turnover of staff who care for the trauma patient. Stress related symptoms are causing increasing levels of sick leave and those individuals affected frequently end up leaving the speciality and even the profession. This personal suffering and loss to the service can be prevented if steps are taken early enough. Trauma nurses assume highly skilled roles to benefit others. They are frequently described as performing extraordinary tasks to resuscitate patients, but this does not alter the fact that trauma nurses remain ordinary people. Stress is a state of physiological and psychological arousal as the result of a threat, challenge or change. Trauma team members respond normally and naturally to protect, maintain and enhance life. Understanding physical, mental and emotional responses can help us to use stress positively and reduce distress. Nurses are in an excellent position to be able to initiate measures to alleviate distress, by acquiring and sharing the necessary technical, human element and supervisory skills. Another excellent way of alleviating distress is by running debriefing or diffusion sessions following difficult resuscitations.

Point for discussion

● Identify signs which may indicate that individual members of the trauma team are suffering as the result of stress.

Advocacy

The vast majority of resources in terms of money, education and research are directed towards the physiological and life-threatening aspects of trauma. However, some of the more lasting effects arise from the emotional damage that trauma has inflicted on patients and their loved ones. In many ways it is easy to justify this direction of resources, as physiological needs are generally more obvious and easy to categorize and clearly psychosocial stability is pointless if the patient is dead. Nevertheless, psychosocial aspects of trauma care must be addressed early if long term damage is to be avoided.

If nurses are to act as the patient's advocate, confrontation with others and potential disagreements are inevitable. This can result in a great deal of additional stress. If the trauma nurse is able to approach interactions with other trauma team members in an assertive way, much of this additional stress could be avoided.

All components of the nurse's role must be woven into the total team effort, aimed at optimal patient outcome.

Point for discussion

● Discuss the benefits of patient advocacy pertaining to trauma.

BRITISH TRAUMA EDUCATION FOR NURSES IN RECENT YEARS

Prior to 1991, no formal education was available for nurses specifically aimed at the care of multiply injured patients. The English National Board Accident and Emergency courses had no obligation to provide instruction concerning trauma care. A survey of A and E nurses in 1991 (Hamilton, 1991) concluded that 46% of 94 nurses questioned had received no specific education in trauma care. The educational opportunities which were available did not reach the more junior nurses, who it appeared would benefit most. It became clear that junior nurses (qualified less than one year) were looking after injured patients more often than the senior nurses who had received education. Hamilton's study suggested that there was urgent need to develop nurse education in this area. Earlier medical recommendations for the management of patients with major injuries (Royal College of Surgeons, 1988) were echoed. The result of not recognizing trauma care as a speciality area was identified, along with requirements for the introduction of specific education at pre- and postgraduate level.

Since the publication of such reports, trauma services and education have become high profile areas in British health care. The government has commissioned comparative studies of specialist trauma services provided in Stoke on Trent with more traditional British services based at Preston Royal Infirmary and Hull Royal Infirmary. The issue is currently undergoing intense scrutiny and there has been a welcome growth of interest from paramedical, nursing and medical specialities. This, combined with the current changes in nurse education at pre- and postregistration level, should ensure that formal education for nurses concerned with caring for the multiply injured patient will be an essential prerequisite to practice in any critical care area receiving injured patients.

Point for discussion

● Why do you think that junior nurses are caring for injured patients more often than specifically trained senior nurses?

OPTIONS FOR TRAUMA NURSE TRAINING

In order to pursue the most appropriate training option, A and E nurses must consider three areas. Firstly, the specific roles of the nurse caring for the multiply injured patient. Trauma nurses assume several different roles, some of which are dependent and interdependent and some of which are independent. These roles must all be clearly identified before suitable training can be commenced.

Secondly, it is essential that any education be based on the same principles as those of other team members. All trauma team members **must** speak the same language.

Thirdly, individual trauma nurses seeking training must identify where their own deficiencies, interests and needs lie, so that training opportunities can be chosen appropriately.

At present in this country, there are three options for trauma nurse training aimed at patient care during the 'golden hour' (Cowley, 1976):

1. Advanced Trauma Nursing Course (ATNC);
2. Trauma Nursing Core Course (TNCC);
3. Advanced Trauma Life Support for physicians (ATLS).

TNCC and ATNC are courses developed for nurses, by nurses. Currently nurses can attend ATLS in an observation capacity only.

The aims of TNCC, ATNC and ATLS are concerned with rapid assessment and resuscitation in a prompt, definitive and standardized way during the 'golden hour' (Buckles, 1990). The ultimate aim is to reduce morbidity and mortality and there is no doubt that the quality and speed of assessment and treatment during the couple of hours following injury influences patient outcome.

ATLS

The ATLs course for physicians was developed in the USA during 1977 when, through personal tragedy, an American surgeon recognized that the trauma system did not work (American College of Surgeons, 1989). The course is run under the auspices of the American College of Surgeons and it is strictly standardized, continually updated and improved. Having been developed over 11 years, ATLS was brought to Britain in November 1988. By the end of 1992, approximately 2500 doctors had been through the ATLS course.

TNCC

TNCC was developed in 1986, also in the USA, and is controlled by the American Emergency Nurses Association (ENA). This course is for nurses only and based on the role of the US emergency department nurse.

The emphasis of TNCC is on team work and the ABCDE approach to multiply injured patient care is applied (ENA, 1988). Once the primary survey is complete and resuscitation is underway, a detailed head to toe survey is commenced to identify all injuries. A sequential, initial rapid assessment is integrated with resuscitation and correction of life-threatening problems.

TNCC was imported into the UK in November 1990. Regardless of previous experience, the first group of TNCC participants declared that they had benefited from the course and that their management of trauma improved following the course (Castille, 1991).

The Emergency Nurses Association (1988) formulated the belief statements from which TNCC was developed:

1. That optimal care of the trauma patient is best accomplished within a framework in which all members of the trauma team use a systematic, standardized approach to the care of the multiply injured patient.
2. Emergency nurses are essential members of the trauma team. Morbidity and mortality of trauma patients can be significantly reduced by educating nurses to competently provide trauma care.
3. The ENA and its constituents have the responsibility to facilitate trauma related continuing educational opportunities for nurses who provide care to trauma patients.

ATNC

Preparatory work for the design of the ATNC began in early 1989. Nurses were beginning to voice concern over attending ATLS courses as observers and being unable to attend as full participants. The Royal College of Nursing and the Royal College of Surgeons of England pledged their firm commitment to shared learning opportunities and supported the creation of ATNC.

The ATNC is based on a set of values and beliefs generated by a group of British trauma nurses, examples of which are that:

- the multiply injured patient has a right to be cared for by a specifically trained nurse;
- shared learning opportunities produce greater team cohesion and mutual understanding of each other's professional roles;

- participants on the course already have existing expertise, skill and knowledge on which to build;
- participants are motivated to learn and are self-directed;
- individuals can complement each other's roles, if aims, objectives and strategies are explicit;
- individuals, through understanding and clarifying their role, are more effective in fulfilling that role.

According to Westaby (1989), the key to effective trauma care lies in uninterrupted and skilful treatment during progression along the therapeutic chain. The efficacy of the therapeutic chain is only as good as its weakest link. It is essential that nurses do not represent this weak link and they must therefore be able to provide skilful care. To provide skilful care, access to specialized training must be available to every nurse who assumes a role within the trauma team.

Point for discussion

● Identify the benefits of undergoing TNCC and ATNC training.

CONTENT OF AVAILABLE COURSES

The ATNC is a five day course which incorporates the two and a half day ATLS course and shared learning with medical colleagues. Nursing participants spend a further two and a half days addressing nursing issues, one and a half days before and one day after ATLS. The 12 nurses and 16 doctors on each joint course have been enthusiastic in their commitment to joint learning and have maintained a clear vision of the aims of ATNC/ATLS: first and foremost, better quality trauma care for the patient and second, the interdependence and mutual respect required to achieve this end.

TNCC is a 2½–3 day course, taking 16 participants. Both TNCC and ATNC content is available in a training manual, which is sent to each participant several weeks before the course for preparatory study. A pretest is also provided before the course, which helps students to prepare for final written assessments. Successful course completion requires a mark of 80% or more on written assessments and a satisfactory performance in all practical skill stations.

Despite the large volume of course content covered in a relatively short time, participants who prepare comprehensively beforehand ultimately do well.

The ATLS course is built upon a dogmatic approach, teaching a simple, safe method of managing the trauma patient. Whilst recognizing that there may be other systems or approaches to trauma care, the ATLS method has been shown to be safe over more than a decade in the USA (Skinner, 1992a).

A major advantage of the ATLS course is that human or sheep cadavers are used to gain experience in the revision of techniques of certain invasive procedures, adding a significant degree of realism and excitement to the course. Nurses join this section to familiarize themselves with anatomical landmarks, required equipment and safe, effective techniques. The objective is not to provide nurses with the skills required to assume expanded roles in the clinical area.

Successful completion of all courses includes success at a 'moulage' station. The moulage station is considered to be the main focus of the course by many and generates a significant level of stress for a high proportion of participants. Some compare the stress of such skills assessments with the anxiety experienced when managing a real patient in the resuscitaiton room (Skinner, 1992b).

An appropriately made up individual, often a nurse or medical student, acts as the trauma victim. Circumstances surrounding the traumatic incident are described to the course participant and for 20–30 minutes, the instructor appraises the candidate's ability to assess and resuscitate the patient using ATNC, ATLS or TNCC principles.

Certification for all courses lasts four years, after which the candidate must repeat all assessments.

Point for discussion

● What method of course assessment would you consider to be most appropriate following trauma training?

Practical skill stations

ATNC

Initial assessment skills
Spinal lifting and turning
Airway management
Venous cutdown
Pericardiocentesis
Chest drain insertion   } Shared learning
Needle cricothyroidotomy   with ATLS colleagues
Surgical cricothyroidotomy
Diagnostic peritoneal lavage

TNCC

Initial assessment skills
Spinal immobilization

Airway management
Multiple trauma intervention
Helmet removal
Splinting

Lecture content

ATNC, ATLS and TNCC

Initial assessment skills
Shock
Thoracic trauma
Abdominal trauma
Head trauma
Spine and spinal cord trauma
Extremity trauma
Burns and cold injury
Stabilization and transport

TNCC only

Epidemiology of trauma and mechanism of injury
Multiple trauma
Eye trauma
Facial trauma
Crisis intervention

ATNC only

The role of the nurse within the trauma team
Burn assessment
Observations and trauma scoring
Psychosocial aspects
How to influence change
Assertiveness skills
Physiological compensatory mechanisms in trauma
Creating a suitable trauma room environment
Medicolegal aspects
Stress associated with trauma team membership

The nursing component of the ATNC is less didactic than the ATLS part of the course. The focus is adjusted to accommodate contributions from and discussion between participants, although specific objectives for each session have been carefully established.

INSTRUCTOR TRAINING

Participants who perform well on the provider courses may be invited to take part in a three day course for instructors.

ATNC/ATLS instructor courses are held at the Royal College of Surgeons of England. Core content of the provider courses is assumed, although retested by multiple choice questionnaire and moulage. Nurses and doctors learn together how to teach others at future ATNC and ATLS courses and are continuously assessed throughout the course by professional educators.

TNCC instructor courses are organized by the TNCC faculty and follow a similar format. The difference is that nurses teach other nurses to teach TNCC.

PLANS FOR THE FUTURE

For the future, the main focus of ATNC, TNCC and ATLS is to increase accessibility for those concerned with trauma care during the 'golden hour', whilst maintaining quality of course content. As courses proliferate around the country, it becomes increasingly difficult to control quality and maintain uniform standards. Strategies will have to be developed to monitor this situation.

Many of those involved in the initial management of trauma and preparation for trauma team roles have become increasingly concerned with trauma team building. Effective team work is essential for quality trauma care; even the most advanced levels of knowledge and skills can be rendered useless if a strong team network is not established. Team building skills are learned skills and must therefore be taught. At their 1991 strategy conference, Cadbury Schweppes sent its managers out to sea, crewing squarerigged sailing ships, with one practical objective: to reinforce its message about team work (Heller, 1992). Perhaps some similar exercise would encourage training team members to work together more effectively.

Finally, when considering the future of all trauma courses, the issue of funding for education and training must be pursued. A significant number of our nursing course participants are self-funding and many are not even granted study leave by their employers. Fortunately, our medical colleagues enjoy comparatively easy access to funding and leave. This is perhaps a sad reflection on the way in which education for nurses is viewed by budget holders. Chiarella (1990) refers to an absence of 'political will' to fund education, hence it is essential that the benefits of education and training are clearly identified and presented in an articulate way. One common excuse is that funds are not available and that all staff are having to 'tighten their belts'.

Well-managed units with well-trained employees keep them and training is one reason why people stay.

Points for discussion

● In what ways can the A and E nurse influence decisions regarding funding for education?

● What measures may be taken to control quality as courses proliferate around the country?

HOW TO APPLY FOR THE COURSES

ATNC: Miss Debbie Wallis
District Resuscitation Training Officer
Bart's City Lifesaver Office
St Bartholomew's Hospital
West Smithfield
London EC1A 7BE

TNCC: Mr Peter Dowds
24 Middlewich Road
Nantwich CW5 6HL

ATLS: Ms Angela Ezekial
The Royal College of Surgeons of England
35–43 Lincoln's Inn Fields
London WC2A 3PN

CONCLUSION

Trauma training in this country is making dramatic inroads into the management of patients with major injuries. The ATNC, TNCC and ATLS courses support the development of a universal language for trauma team members, which in turn promotes the establishment of united and effective trauma teams.

Clearly, it is time to commit ourselves to a programme aimed at training any health care worker who comes into contact with the multiply injured patient.

Nurses, by the very nature of their role, are intimately involved in the initial assessment and resuscitation of trauma victims. However, trauma teams can consist of many individuals: prehospital personnel, porters, medical and radiography staff to name but a few. Some of our colleagues may need support in pressing for better training and education for themselves.

By the end of 1992, there were 126 ATNC trained nurses and 24 instructors, which means that, at an estimate, there are a further 1700 active A and E nurses to be trained if we are to provide 24-hour cover in all British A and E departments receiving multiply injured patients.

REFERENCES

American College of Surgeons (1989) Advanced Trauma Life Support Programme, Committee on Trauma, American College of Surgeons, Illinois.

Anderson, I.D., Woodford, M., de Dombal, F.T. and Irving, M. (1988) Retrospective study of 1000 trauma deaths from injury in England and Wales. *British Medical Journal*, 296, 1305–8.

Buckles, E. (1990) Advanced trauma life support. *Nursing Standard*, 28(4), 54–5.

Carl, L. and Champion, H.R. (1986) Optimal resuscitation unit design, in *Trauma Nursing: Principles and Practice*, (ed. B.A. Kenezevitch), Appleton-Century-Crofts, Norwalk, CT.

Castille, K. (1991) Trauma training for nurses. *Nursing*, 4(32), 22–3.

Chiarella, M. (1990) Developing the credibility of continuing education. *Nurse Education Today*, 10, 70–3.

Cowley, R.A. (1976) The resuscitation and stabilisation of major multiple trauma; patients in a trauma centre environment. *Clinical Medicine*, 83, 14.

Davies, S. (1993) Trauma scoring. *Accident and Emergency Nursing*, 1(3), 125–31.

Department of Health (1992) *The Health of the Nation*, HMSO, London.

Emergency Nurses Association (1988) *Trauma Nursing Core Course Manual*, Award Printing Corporation, Illinois.

Glasser, W. (1989) Communication, in *Nurse Manager: A Systems Approach*, (ed. D.A. Gilies), W.B. Saunders, Philadelphia.

Hadfield, L.V. (1992) *Advanced Trauma Nursing Course Manual* (unpublished)

Hadfield, L.V. (1993) Preparation for the nurse as part of the trauma team. *Accident and Emergency Nursing*, 1(3), 154–60.

Halpern, J.S. (1987) *The Nurse as Part of the Trauma Team*, Bronson Management Services Corporation, Michigan.

Hamilton, A. (1991) Trauma training. *Nursing Times*, 87(2), 42–4.

Heller, R. (1992) Why getting into training is a must. *Business Life*, **May**, 16–20.

Myers, M. and Hopperstead, L. (1982) Advanced trauma life support for physicians and nurses: a pilot programme. *Journal of Emergency Nursing*, 8(3), 123–6.

Office of Population, Censuses and Surveys (1991) *OPCS Monitor*, Series DH4, No. 91/2, HMSO, London.

Royal College of Surgeons of England (1988) *Report of the Working Party on the Management of Patients with Major Injuries*, RCS, London.

Skinner, D. (1992a) *The Advanced Trauma Life Support Course*, Royal London Hospital Emergency Medical Service, London.

Skinner, D. (1992b) Advanced trauma life support. *Care of the Critically Ill*, 8(3), 98–9.

Trauma Nursing Coalition (1992) Resource Document for Nursing Care of the Trauma Patient (unpublished).

Westaby, S. (1989) Trauma: the problem and some solutions, in *Trauma: Pathogenesis and Treatment*, (ed. S. Westaby), Heinemann, Oxford.

World Health Organization (1989) *World Health Statistics Annual*, WHO, Geneva.

Yates, D.W., Woodford, M. and Hollis, S. (1992) Preliminary analysis of the care of injured patients in 33 British hospitals: first report of the United Kingdom major trauma outcome study. *British Medical Journal*, **305**, 737–40.

CHAPTER 5

An introduction to quality issues in the A and E department

J. Dutton

INTRODUCTION

Everyone has a definition for quality for it is a word attached to just about every aspect of nursing. This chapter is concerned with definitions of quality and ways in which quality initiatives may be applied within the A and E department. A theme running through the chapter is that of perceptions in relation to quality. Previous experience or prior expectations may influence the ways in which staff and patients view quality. This may result in different expectations and understandings of the service as provided by A and E staff and used by patients, their families and friends.

The organization of the chapter sets the scene for the reader. An overview of quality initiatives relevant to A and E including an introduction to total quality management is provided. The presence of a number of concepts serves as an introduction to quality as an issue which demands further analysis and debate by the reader.

The reader is invited to consider the content of the chapter within their own area of clinical practice through the use of discussion points. The intended outcome of this is to encourage the reader to determine the most appropriate approach to quality in relation to the resources available within their own A and E department. It should be noted that although various paths to addressing quality issues are provided within this chapter, there are no ready answers. The reader may need to seek out information from their own clients to help establish questions and answers. Establishing customer response to service delivery requires the adequate design of tools such as questionnaires. Within the chapter guidance is provided to help readers design questionnaires for such a task.

Finally information within this chapter has been organized in sections which are designed to be dipped into or read in relation to other sections of the chapter or book. The reference list at the end of the chapter supplies further reading for those wishing to develop further ideas put forward within the text.

DEFINITIONS

A patient's perception of quality care in A and E may be that he is able to drink a cup of tea before going to theatre wearing his own clothes. A nurse's perception of quality care in the same situation may focus around adequate psychosocial and physical preparation of the patient for his forthcoming operation. Kemp and Richardson (1990) argue that quality can only be conceived in terms of the goodness which is inherent in the object with which we are concerned. Deer (1989) states that 'Quality in health care is a lot less easy to describe than to lament when it isn't there'.

The *Concise Oxford English Dictionary* (1987) defines quality as 'a degree of excellence'. Oakland (1990) simply explains quality as meaning 'meeting the requirements'. He argues that the requirements are of paramount importance in the assessment of quality. If we find out what these requirements are and how they can be achieved and maintained then we can slowly begin to understand quality.

WHAT IS QUALITY?

If we can agree that quality is meeting the requirements then it is important that A and E staff consider the following.

1. Who their customers are;
2. The true requirements/needs of their customers;
3. How they can continually meet these needs;
4. How they can measure whether they are meeting the needs;
5. How to monitor changes in needs.

While it can be argued that patients or clients are the customers of health care, Pfeffer (1992) uses the term 'institutional customers' to describe general practitioner fundholders, resource managers, care managers, purchasers of health care and contract holders in competitive tendering. Pfeffer (1992) states that if the true requirements of these customers are not continually met then they can vote with their feet – an extremely negative but effective customer response to service delivery.

In considering the five points on page 89, A and E departments should be striving towards providing a quality driven service. If this strategy is adopted throughout a hospital or health care organization, then it is often described as total quality management. Hosking (1992) explains this concept as 'a documented set of defined activities and events serving to implement the quality system in an organization'.

Historically most health care services have evolved as demand led services. However, demand does not always reflect the greatest needs of the client and services responsive only to demand may be inappropriate or inadequate in relation to needs.

Points for discussion

● How would you define quality in relation to A and E care?

● Who is the client or customer in A and E?

● Who purchases A and E services in your hospital setting? For example, are general practitioners purchasers of A and E services?

● Is your A and E service demand led or are the true requirements of the customer considered?

QUALITY COMMITMENT

In order to meet the true requirements of the customer A and E departments should see quality assurance as an integral part of the overall programme of health care delivery. It should be a dynamic, continuous, permanent part of every health professional's regular activities.

Deer (1989) writes that:

> Quality is not a destination at which you arrive but a journey during which the steps of establishing objectives, developing strategies, executing tasks and evaluating the results need to be trod again and again.

This dynamism and process of continuous improvement in meeting the needs of the customer can only be achieved through the commitment of all members of the organization. Oakland (1990) explains that every part, every activity, every person in a company affects and is in turn affected by others. For health care to be truly effective, every single part of it must work properly together. Nowhere is this more apparent than in the multidisciplinary environment of an A and E department. Total quality management (TQM) is seen as an approach to improving the whole organization by involving the whole organization. If every individual in the A and E setting worked properly together and recognized that every activity affects and in turn is affected by others then there would be a widespread improvement in the quality of care delivery to patients. TQM allows for this philosophy to become reality. A total quality commitment spanning all levels and all disciplines is what is required if A and E departments wish to meet the true requirements of its customers.

Koch (1991) lists features of TQM including standard setting, monitoring and review, quality of information production, customer feedback strategies and action, training for quality, communication, resource management and integration of quality criteria into contracts. The need for quality in health care has in the past been bureaucratically administered by a quality strategy being agreed by a group of health care experts. A quality team was then appointed to ensure the strategy accomplished its aim. While it is necessary to adopt a positive management culture committed to providing quality service, staff at all levels must be encouraged to produce quality improvements in their own particular services and be responsible for achieving and further developing those improvements.

Points for discussion

● How could the staff in your A and E department work more closely together to maximize their effectiveness?

● Who is *responsible* for quality in your A and E department?

● How could total quality management be introduced into your hospital setting?

While there is a need to ensure the total quality management approach is coordinated throughout the health care services, the role of a quality assurance team should be primarily one of facilitator and coordinator not, as is commonly the case, one which focuses on inspection, measurement and criticism. Individual staff or a bureaucratic department being identified as responsible for quality often results in the organization believing that quality issues are being addressed by someone else and that there is no need for them to consider quality. This passive approach can be counter-productive and can result in an isolated quality assurance department who are only able to perform the inspect, measure and criticize functions.

In order to meet the true requirements of the customer, A and E department staff must ensure that quality is a dynamic, continuous and permanent part of their regular activities. Quality assurance experts should be appointed to coordinate quality strategies and facilitate changes beneficial to staff and patients, but staff at grassroots level should be directly involved and responsible for quality care in the A and E setting.

Through reorganization of health care management, medical and nursing staff now appear to have more of an active role in the management of their services. Responsible purchasers, for example district health authorities, are acknowledging that quality measures, standards and successful outcomes are an essential part of contract specification. At last, the service is realizing that purchasing is not just about an assessment of the nature and quality of services required and the order of practices. Ham (1992) states that 'Contracts are a key mechanism in the (quality) process, offering an opportunity to set out more explicitly than in the past, the quality of care that should be delivered to patients'. The White Paper *Working for Patients* (DoH, 1989) states that 'Contracts will need to spell out clearly what is required for each hospital in terms of the price, quality and the nature of service to be provided. A hospital which fails to meet the terms of a contract will risk losing patients and revenue'.

Points for discussion

- What quality strategies are employed at a district level and at an A and E departmental level?

- Is quality care provision considered in the contract specification for your A and E department's services?

QUALITY APPLICATIONS IN ACCIDENT AND EMERGENCY

As previously addressed, for any quality system to be effective in A and E it must be seen as continuous, permanent and dynamic; dynamic because health care needs are always changing, reflecting changes in technology and in society; continuous and permanent because it is essential that A and E staff equate quality with these concepts to encourage total commitment to quality and a sense of ownership for the success of the quality applications. At present, quality applications in A and E appear to be developing through single disciplines.

In the A and E situation there is an abundance of disciplines, tasks, skills and quality issues which require effective coordination to function successfully and efficiently. Ultimately, any quality system in A and E should be planned, implemented and evaluated across all the disciplines involved in A and E care or service support. Total quality management, multiagency meetings and multidisciplinary audit are methods which attempt to address this. Currently, the main approaches to quality issues which are directly or indirectly addressed across the disciplines appear to be quality circles (Peters and Waterman, 1991) and multidisciplinary meetings. Other applications which can be used to address quality in A and E include patient satisfaction questionnaires, retrospective review of complaints, quality standards and single discipline audits. This chapter will continue by discussing these applications in more detail.

QUALITY CIRCLES

The quality circle is an imported Japanese concept which has been used in British industry since the 1970s. Peters and Waterman (1991) state that quality circles can be a gimmick allowing management to be comfortable in the knowledge that a quality tool is being used without having to actually *do the job of real people involvement*.

Quality circles operate by employees brainstorming specific issues pertaining to their work situation. They take responsibility for suggesting innovative quality improvements, identifying and recommending solutions to problems and, with management approval, acting on those recommendations. This ultimately results in improved productivity for the organization.

Bryant and Kearns (1982) conclude that two main conditions are necessary for the success of quality circles: *workers who are willing to participate and managers who are willing to let them*. Quality circles can operate very effectively in A and E. Not only can effective practical improvements be made but communication across the disciplines can be enhanced and a more understanding working relationship can be achieved as a result.

Point for discussion

● What issues would you like to be addressed using quality circles in your A and E department?

PATIENT SATISFACTION QUESTIONNAIRES

Satisfaction questionnaires are generally employed to assess the consumer response to the delivery of care. In A and E departments, this type of survey is seen as a quick and easy way to capture the views of the patient in an easy to interpret format. Unfortunately, unless the questionnaire is extremely well designed, the resulting data can be meaningless.

Point for discussion

● How useful is the knowledge that, for example, 50% of respondents attending the department on 1st March were 'unhappy' with the reception area? Why were they 'unhappy', what does unhappy mean, does it mean the same to everyone, what part of the reception area were they unhappy about – clerical system, triage, seating arrangement or the refreshment availability?

When designing a questionnaire, every question must be critically examined. The main points to consider when selecting or developing a questionnaire are:

- Identify key individuals to assist in the questionnaire development.
- Identify the essential content to be covered.
- Search the literature for previous examples of questionnaires which match what you are hoping to achieve.
- Identify the target groups you wish to complete the questionnaire.
- Carefully plan the order of the questionnaire items.
- Include the instructions on how to mark responses on the questionnaire.
- Consider the need for a covering letter to accompany the questionnaire.
- Perform a pilot test of the questionnaire.
- Ensure questionnaire validity and reliability.
- Consider and decide the most effective way to analyse the data.

(Burns and Grove, 1987)

If the A and E department finances the patient satisfaction survey then consultancy support can be purchased to assist with design, distribution and analysis of the questionnaire.

Point for discussion

● What essential content would you identify for inclusion in an A and E department patient satisfaction questionnaire?

COMPLAINTS REVIEW

Well-designed patient satisfaction questionnaires are an effective way to monitor whether the consumer is satisfied with the A and E service provided. Close examination of consumer complaints can generate equally valuable information. The *NHS Handbook* (Connah and Lancaster, 1989), states that 'Complaints can be used as a stimulus for improvements in service delivery and a vehicle for developing staff'.

Pfeffer (1992) argues that 'While systems of redress and complaint are important, they discriminate against the most vulnerable, the people who lack the necessary confidence, time, energy and resources to pursue a grievance'.

A review of seven years of complaints in a British inner city A and E department was conducted by Hunt and Glucksman (1991). In summarizing, they stated that the most common complaints were those regarding attitude, missed diagnosis, waiting time, cursory examination and poor communication. They also noted that all the above causes of complaint were 'amenable to improvement'. This work highlights the benefits which can be gained by close examination of complaints received. Unbiased examination of the circumstances of each complaint received by the A and E department can result in a systematic evaluation of work practices and service provision.

Point for discussion

● How can complaints be used constructively in your A and E department to stimulate improvements in the service?

QUALITY STANDARDS

A standard is defined by the *Concise Oxford English Dictionary* (1987) as 'a weight or measure to which others conform and by which the accuracy or quality of others is judged'.

Sale (1990) writes on the need to identify standards and criteria in order to establish the quality of nursing service. However, Shelley (1992) cautions that 'to produce a comprehensive quality manual the standards it contains tend to be written in stone'. This means that every time there is a change in practice, the manual has to be rewritten, making the whole process cumbersome and bureaucratic. Ervin *et al.* (1989) write that if quality is concerned with meeting the customer's requirements then standards should be seen as written evidence of those requirements.

A and E departments need to decide agreed quality standards of service delivery which best meet the true identified requirements of the customer. This is an enormous task fraught with difficulties especially in ensuring that the standards are desirable and acceptable when used as a measure of quality provision. Kemp and Richardson (1990), writing within the arena of standard setting for nursing, state that standards should be 'measurable, realistic, appropriate, desirable, acceptable and unambiguous'.

Donabedian's (1966) 'structure, process, outcome' method of organizing health care delivery has been chosen by many health care professionals for organizing quality standards. Donabedian's framework is not, however, the only method and health professionals concerned with preparing standards should at least be aware of this fact. Kerr and Trantow (1969) identified components of care, sites of care and the amounts and timeliness of care as the three areas which could be examined to evaluate the quality of the interaction. An economic model was suggested by Heggerty (1970) including health status, medical needs, demand, manpower, capital, training, utilization and supply facilities.

Kitson (1989) describes the theoretical framework for quality assurance in health care developed by the Royal College of Nursing (RCN) Standards of Care Project, using Donabedian's 'structure, process, outcome' approach at an organizational, professional and individual level. The persons compiling the standards can encounter real problems in the interpretation of the terms **structure, process** and **outcome**. An individual's position within the organization will undoubtedly determine what they consider as structure, process and outcome. On standards and specification, Oakland (1990) writes, 'To fulfil their purpose, they must be written in terminology which is understood and in a manner which is unambiguous and so cannot be the subject of differing interpretation'.

Sale (1990) suggests that ward staff write standards on topics they select. Sale describes these as local standards and continues by discussing the need for universal or generic standards and district standards.

Points for discussion

● Are standard statements available for all areas of patient care in your A and E department?

● Are the standards reviewed periodically to ensure they are reflective of good practice based on current research?

● If local standards are developed, do they reflect the true requirements of the consumer or do they reflect the level of quality which the A and E department considers achievable?

QUALITY AUDIT

The *Concise Oxford English Dictionary* (1987) defines audit as 'an official examination (of accounts)'. Oakland (1990) described quality audit and review as 'one method in general use for checking the system'. He states that quality audits and review 'subject each area of an organization's activity to a systematic critical examination, every component of the total system being included'.

According to Oakland, the aim of a quality audit should be to disclose the strengths and weaknesses and the main areas of vulnerability or risk. While some quality audit tools attempt to examine comprehensively all the components of a service, audits are often designed to address clinical or organizational components of health care delivery via a single discipline. In A and E, medical staff commonly identify audit as a retrospective review of their clinical practice either by case discussion with peers on selected patients or patient types or by a more formal planned programme of review of selected patient groups. Through review, discussion and constructive criticism, this style of audit often elicits improved quality of medical practice.

A quality audit in professions allied to medicine often reflects the medical style of audit as described above: systematic retrospective reviews of practice based on a set number of indicators. Nursing quality audit has, until recently, been extremely difficult to implement in A and E as no comprehensive tool was available designed specifically for this purpose. Nurses have employed various methods of quality examination, including questioning the patient via patient satisfaction questionnaires, ideas boxes, questioning the staff, quality circles, quality improvement schemes and rewarding quality initiatives. While all these methods can be effective in examining and improving the quality of nursing care they cannot be considered a systematic, critical examination of nursing activity, i.e. quality audit.

The Kings Fund's *Organizational Audit* (1990) provides quality criteria for examination of the organizational activities of an A and E department. It is an invaluable tool to be used in the process of quality audit allowing service providers to identify areas of weakness and shortfall in the organization of the service. Certain criteria require the professional judgement of the auditor and therefore could result in some subjectivity.

One example of a specific organizational style audit is the updating of the A and E record as described by Casserly and Tomas (1992). Eight records in use in six A and E departments in the Mersey region were reviewed. The structure of the record, the printed matter and the designated areas for documentation by the administrators, nursing and medical staff were studied in addition to the advantages of the record when referring patients to other hospital departments and the application of computers in collecting and handling data.

Ultimately, a multidisciplinary quality audit tool is what is required for any A and E department. This will provide comprehensive, valid and reliable audit of the overall quality of care which A and E departments provide for their patients. When single discipline audits and organizational audits have been further refined for use in the A and E situation they can be adapted for use as contributors to such a comprehensive multidisciplinary audit tool.

ACCIDENT AND EMERGENCY NURSING QUALITY AUDIT

Goldstone and Dutton (1992) describe *Accident and Emergency Monitor* as an audit of the quality of nursing care in A and E departments. This chapter will continue by describing the research and development of the audit tool.

In 1990, the need was recognized for the development of a practical set of audit criteria relevant to nursing care delivery to patients and relatives in A and E departments. A research assistant post was established enabling the researcher to work as part-time research assistant and part-time A and E sister. A second research assistant post for an overlapping period of 12 months was established at Leeds Polytechnic. The project commenced in June 1990 and resulted in the publication in November 1991 *of Accident and Emergency Monitor* (Dutton *et al.*, 1991), an audit of the quality of nursing care in A and E departments.

Monitor (Goldstone *et al.*, 1983) style audit tools are the most widely used and most comprehensive audit tools available designed specifically for audit of quality of nursing care delivery in the United Kingdom. Monitor is an adaptation and development for the UK of the Rush Medicus nursing process methodology (Haussman *et al.*, 1976). Using Monitor enables care given to be assessed and the attention of the user can easily focus on areas of competence and areas requiring improvement. Minimum professional judgement is required for the questions to be answered. A yes/no response is required for observable aspects of quality care. The documentation provided enables an index on a scale of 0–100 to be calculated for the quality of care delivered. This index is the percentage of the questions coded as 'yes'. Monitor style audit tools have now been developed for most specialities. They all share a question format requiring yes/no responses and a similar response grid layout.

The research assistants gained theoretical and practical knowledge of Monitor based on implementation of the Monitor audit tools *Junior Monitor* (Galvin and Goldstone, 1988) and *Senior Monitor* (Goldstone and Maselino-Okai, 1986) and, in liaison with other researchers, engaged in compiling *Health Visiting Monitor* (Whitaker and Goldstone, 1991) and *Equal If* for persons with learning difficulties (Cumming and Goldstone, 1991).

In order to compile a viable, applicable and valid document for use in A and E nursing nationally, the previously used Monitor development protocols indicated that up to six working parties in contrasting health authorities might suggest or brainstorm relevant criteria. These working parties comprised 4–5 clinically based A and E nurses identified by the managers as ideal role models. The working parties brainstormed quality criteria over a six month period using patient vignettes. By informal interpretation of conversation and language many quality criteria were described and recorded. Following refinement of the criteria by parallel discussion in subsequent health authorities, a master list of criteria was generated. A detailed literature search was conducted with relatively unproductive results.

Therefore, in order to ascertain precise details of nursing care systems in use in the UK a self-completion questionnaire was sent to every A and E department in the UK and the Republic of Ireland. The aim of the survey was to gain a comprehensive overview of how nursing care is taught, assessed, planned, implemented and evaluated in the 314 units addressed. 233 questionnaires were returned giving a 71% response, of which 97% wished to be kept informed of developments regarding the research. Figure 5.1 shows the major issues featured in the questionnaire. Items 6, 7, 8, 9, 10, 11 and 12 gave positive **yes** responses of less than 50% in each case. Of those units (30%) which claimed to have a way of assessing the quality of care, only 47% could give a description of their way which included quality circles, audit, departmental meetings and patient satisfaction surveys.

Of those units (48%) which claimed to use a triage system, only 27% responded positively to the request to send details of policies, documentation and teaching relevant to the system. Although 45% of units claimed to use the nursing process, less than half of these (40%) supplied even brief details of documentation and of the 29% which had written standards of care, only 27% could offer details and examples.

All the data collected as a result of this questionnaire indicate that the quality of nursing care was not being addressed comprehensively in A and E departments. The need for nursing staff to be able to use a quality tool which is specifically designed for use in A and E departments was further reinforced.

This initial questionnaire study proved invaluable as a source of reference, provider of information and starting point for the development of *Accident and Emergency Monitor* (Dutton *et al.*, 1991). Quality audit criteria development needed to consider all the issues addressed in the initial survey study. The overall design or structure of *Accident and Emergency Monitor* would clearly not be based around any single issue or model.

In February 1990 the Royal College of Nursing Accident and Emergency Association provided funding for a second researcher. This

Question	Yes %	No %	Looking into it %
1. Do you run an ENB 199 course in Accident and Emergency nursing?	9	84	6
2. Do you have a local RCN A and E forum?	73	27	
3. Do you run an ENB course in Accident and Emergency nursing for enrolled nurses?	3	97	
4. Do you provide a specific in-service training for your Accident and Emergency staff?	73	26	
5. Do you provide a specific in-service information/documentation package for your Accident and Emergency staff?	53	40	3
6. Do you have a way of assessing the quality of care in your Accident and Emergency department?	30	62	8
7. Do you have a triage system in operation in your department?	48	46	6
8. Do you apply a nursing model to the care given?	32	64	4
9. Do you use the nursing process in your department?	45	50	5
10. Do you have primary nursing in your Accident and Emergency department?	18	81	
11. Do you have a nurse practitioner system in your department?	9	84	7
12. Does your department have written standards of care?	29	55	16

Sample size: 314 A and E departments in UK and Republic of Ireland. Responses included above for 223 responding departments (71%).

Figure 5.1 Results of survey of nursing practice in A and E departments up to December 1989.

work approached the development of criteria set quite independently. The researcher concentrated on examination of relevant quality criteria available from the *Psychiatric Nursing Monitor* (Goldstone and Doggett, 1990). Reference to the original Rush Medicus (Haussman *et al.*, 1976) developments was used to inform the selection of audit items. A brainstorming session between the three authors then produced an agreed set of criteria for further testing for validity and practicality.

Members of the working parties met once the initial phase of the research was completed in order to contrast, compare and discuss the criteria and ideas resulting from it and revise the master list of criteria. The list of criteria was then sent to a panel of clinical nurses in 140 A and E departments which in the initial survey had expressed interest in this. The 70 random questions were sent to each of the 140 A and E departments involved. Nurses were asked to make face and content validity checks using a five point validity rating scale where 1 represents maximum validity as a quality criterion and 5 represents irrelevance for each criterion.

The data from this validation exercise were analysed and an overwhelmingly positive response was noted, almost all questions meriting a validity score of 1 or 2 with those few scoring 3, 4 or 5 being reconsidered, reworded or omitted. The revised, validated master list was then put through a practical pilot test in five A and E departments. This forms a judgemental sample offering operating characteristics representative of all UK health authority A and E departments.

The final event was a seminar held in December 1990 for all practical participants to discuss results of the piloting exercise and make final amendments to the criteria set. This seminar also considered an additional component of the *Accident and Emergency Monitor* for short stay A and E wards, based on modification of the existing Monitor for medical and surgical units.

As a result of literature analysis, discussion, brainstorming and field testing of the developed *Accident and Emergency Monitor* quality audit tool, two master lists of quality related criteria grouped under three main headings were compiled, one for the unit and one for an associated short stay ward. Each is constructed as follows.

Patient care

This audits and records the care of up to 30 patients and their relatives in an A and E department or ward setting. Included in this section are add-on subsections for minor injury patients and for the care of children under 16 years of age in the unit.

Unit management

This audits the management of a single A and E dpeartment or short stay ward.

Unit profile

This describes the A and E department or ward, including its facilities and resources.

Accident and Emergency Monitor is complete and self-contained and may be used by any A and E department without external help or consultations. A and E departments using *Accident and Emergency Monitor* should find it a useful step in the process of quality assurance. It should serve as a reminder on issues and practice for which quality standards need documenting. It should also be an agent of change, providing as it does a series of pointers to areas which need attention, education or specific resolution.

Subsequent work which will improve the A and E quality audit system and help with its implementation will require further funding.

A and E department staff should ensure quality is written into every agenda if they wish to claim commitment to providing a quality driven service which maintains effective services of appropriate quality within available resources and in accordance with agreed policies.

Sale (1990) recognizes many advantages of using Monitor style audit tools, including providing ward and unit staff with an indicator of the quality of care provided. Sale does, however, identify disadvantages with the Monitor style audit tools, stating that it requires a team of trained auditors to monitor the ward or unit 'which obviously has resource and cost implications for the service'. Sale also states that there are problems with observer reliability and subjective interpretation of the criteria.

The majority of criticism levelled at the Monitor audit tools regards the implementation process, not the audit tool itself. If the audit tool is implemented using the steps suggested by the authors, then few difficulties should occur. Auditor preparation and criteria refinement for local needs are essential if the audit is to be effective and valid.

Point for discussion

● What would be the benefit to the staff and patients in your A and E department of implementing the A and E Monitor quality audit tool?

THE FUTURE FOR QUALITY

One major barrier to improving or assessing quality appears to be the cost in time, money and resources of performing quality audit. The proposed benefits gained from performing the audit must be clearly stated in order to justify the audit costs. Similarly, the initial costs of implementing a total quality management system may seem unnecessary in the current cost conscious health care climate. However, as discussed previously, allowing A and E department staff to adopt a proactive quality conscious culture will undoubtedly produce benefits for the organization in terms of input, throughput and

Patient's Code or Initials	□□□□□□□□□□□□□□□ □□□□□□□□□□□□□□□
Source of information	

Ask patient/ observe	**Is the use of equipment explained to the patient and relatives in a way that they understand?** To patient: I see that you have a _____ . Has someone explained what this is and why you need it, in a clear way that you understand?
Yes No N/A Score	□□□□□□□□□□□□□□□ □□□□□□□□□□□□□□□□ □□□□□□□□□□□□□□□□ □□□□□□□□□□□□□□□□□

Observe/ Ask patient	**Do the nurses listen to the patient?** (To the patient: When you ask questions or make comments do you feel the nurses listen to you and show an interest in what you say?)
Yes No N/A Score	□□□□□□□ □□□□□□□ □□□□□□□□ □□□□□□□□

Ask patient/ relatives/ observe	**If the patient/relative must wait, are they informed why?** Question may be put at any time patient/relatives are waiting. Ask: Do you know why you are waiting? Score 'yes' if informed why waiting and what they are waiting for.
Yes No N/A Score	□□□□□□□□□□□□ □□□□□□□□□□□□□ □□□□□□□□□□□□□ □□□□□□□□□□□□□□

Observe patient/ ask nurse	**If the patient has special communication needs, are these identified and met? (includes interpreters, sign language, etc.)** To nurse: Does Mr/Mrs/Miss _____ have any special communication needs? If no, code N/A unless patient has need identified by auditor, in which case code 'no'. If nurse has identified need, ask: How are these needs met?
Yes No N/A Score	□□□□□□ □□□□□□□ □□□□□□□ □□□□□□□□

The boxes in the above five sections should each extend to 30 units

Figure 5.2 An example of the response grid and audit style (reprinted by kind permission of the *British Journal of Nursing*).

output. Professor Berwick (1992) states that British health care is embarking on a 'new wave of review, accountability and measurement'. He advises that an overall system for quality improvement is adopted. Target 31 of the World Health Organization European Region, Health for All (Connah and Lancaster, 1989) states that 'By 1990 all member states should have built effective mechanisms for ensuring quality of patient care within their health care systems'.

A high level of quality care provision can only be achieved through involvement and commitment from all staff involved in patient care delivery in the A and E department.

Providing a quality driven service can be rewarding and motivating. Andrea and Gross (1991) stress that the provision of the required resources is important in ensuring improvement in care. It is of little benefit auditing the level of care provision and making recommendations if staff are then unable to act on those recommendations due to lack of resources.

Mechanisms are now available allowing A and E departments to comprehensively address quality care provision. No longer do staff have to use the number of new patient attenders each year as an indicator of their importance or effectiveness in the ranks of A and E care.

A and E departments will benefit from addressing quality from a multidisciplinary perspective. Ultimately, a multidisciplinary quality audit tool designed specifically for use in A and E is necessary in order to provide a comprehensive, valid and reliable audit of the overall quality of care which A and E departments provide for their patients.

Quality in A and E should be a dynamic process involving every member of the A and E team. This chapter has attempted to illustrate this and to encourage consideration and reflection on quality related issues and their application in the A and E environment.

Points for discussion

- Does your A and E department have effective mechanisms for ensuring the quality of patient care?

- Does your hospital have effective mechanisms for ensuring the quality of patient care?

- If these mechanisms are not effective, what measures can be taken to improve their effectiveness?

REFERENCES

Andrea, J. and Gross, D. (1991) Comprehensive quality assurance in a level II trauma center emergency department. *Journal of Emergency Nursing*, **17**(3), 137–45.

Berwick, D. (1992) cited in Miller, B. Never mind the quality – look at the value. *Health Service Journal*, **102**(5295), 15.

Bryant, S. and Kearns, J. (1982) Workers' brains as well as their bodies. Quality circles in a federal facility. *Public Administration Review*, **42**(2), 144–50.

Burns, N. and Grove, S.K. (1987) *The Practice of Nursing Research. Conduct, Critique and Utilization*, W.B. Saunders, Philadelphia.

Casserly, H.B. and Tomas, P. (1992) Updating the accident and emergency record. *Injury*, **23**(3), 174–6.

Concise Oxford Dictionary (1987) 7th edition, Oxford University Press, Oxford.

Connah, B. and Lancaster, S. (1989) *NHS Handbook*, 4th edn, National Association of Health Authorities/Macmillan Press Ltd, London.

Cumming, M. and Goldstone, L.A. (1991) *Equal If – Evaluation of Quality in the Management of Mental Handicap Services*, Gale Centre Publications, Loughton, Essex.

Deer, B. (1989) *The Best of Health – Quality and Service*, pp. 7–13, Sunday Times Publication, London.

Department of Health (1989) *Working for Patients*, HMSO, London.

Donabedian, A. (1966) *Evaluating the Quality of Medical Care. Milbank Memorial Fund Quarterly*, **44**(2), 166–206.

Dutton, J.M., Grylls, S.L. and Goldstone, L.A. (1991) *Accident and Emergency Monitor: An Audit of the Quality of Nursing Care in Hospital Accident and Emergency Departments*, Gale Centre Publications, Loughton, Essex.

Ervin, N.E., Chen Shu-Pi, C. and Upshaw, H. (1989) Development of a public health nursing quality assessment measure. *Quality Research Bulletin*, **May**, 138–43.

Galvin, J. and Goldstone, L.A. (1988) *Junior Monitor*, Newcastle-upon-Tyne Polytechnic Products Ltd, Newcastle-upon-Tyne.

Goldstone, L.A., Ball, J.A. and Collich, M.M. (1983) *Monitor – An Index of the Quality of Nursing Care for Acute Medical and Surgical Wards*, Newcastle-upon-Tyne Polytechnic Products Ltd, Newcastle-upon-Tyne.

Goldstone, L.A. and Doggett, D. (1990) *Psychiatric Nursing Monitor: A Quality Assurance Audit for Psychiatric Nursing Care*, Gale Centre Publications, Loughton, Essex.

Goldstone, L.A. and Dutton, J. (1992) Accident and emergency audit. *Nursing*, **15**(1), 26–9.

Goldstone, L.A. and Maselino-Okai, C.V. (1986) *Senior Monitor*, Newcastle-upon-Tyne Polytechnic Products Ltd, Newcastle-upon-Tyne.

Ham, C. (1992) Contract culture. *Health Service Journal*, **102**(5301), 22–4.

Haussman, R.K. Hegyvary, D., Sev, T. and Newman, J.F. (1976) *Monitoring Quality of Nursing Care Part II: Assessment and Study of Correlates*, (DHEW Publications No. (HRA) 86–7), Department of Health, Education and Welfare, Washington DC.

Heggerty, R.J. (1970) Science and ambulatory health services for children. *American Journal of Diseases in Childhood*, **119**, 36–44.

Hosking, J. (1992) Determining the standards: quality assurance. *Nursing*, **5**(1), 24–5.

Hunt, M.T. and Glucksman, M.E. (1991) A review of 7 years of complaints in an inner city accident and emergency department. *Archives of Emergency Medicine*, **8**, 17–23.

Kemp, N. and Richardson, E. (1990) *Quality Assurance in Nursing Practice*, Butterworth Heinemann, Oxford.

Kerr, M. and Trantow, D.J. (1969) Defining, measuring and assessing the quality of health services. *Public Health Reports*, **84**, 415–24.

King's Fund Centre (1990) *Organisational Audit. Accreditation UK; Standards for an Acute Hospital*, King's Fund Centre, London, pp. 124–38.

Kitson, A.L. (1989), *Standard of Care. A Framework for Quality*, Royal College of Nursing Standards of Care Project, Hamilton Press, Middlesex.

Koch, H.V. (1991) Supplying what the 'customer' wants on time. *International Journal of Health Care Quality Assurance*, **3**(6), 3.

Oakland, J.S. (1990) *Total Quality Management*, Heinemann Professional Publishing Ltd, Oxford.

Peters, T.J. and Waterman, R.H. Jr (1991) *In Search of Excellence. Lessons from America's Best Run Companies*, Harper Collins, Glasgow.

Pfeffer, N. (1992) Strings attached. *Health Service Journal*, **102**(5296), 22–3.

Sale, D. (1990) *Quality Assurance. The Essentials of Nursing Management*, Macmillan Education Ltd, Basingstoke.

Shelley, H. (1992), Mission impossible? Standard setting. *Nursing Times*, **88**(16), 37.

Whitaker, C. and Goldstone, L.A. (1991), *Health Visiting Monitor: An Audit of the Quality of Health Visiting Services*, Gale Centre Publications, Loughton, Essex.

CHAPTER 6

Technology in the A and E department: a nursing perspective

J. Dutton

INTRODUCTION

Technology colours the way we all think and live and that applies within the A and E department where all grades of staff and patients have been exposed to varying degrees of technology including information technology.

In the past unrealistic expectations, inadequate consultation, impulsive purchases and poor evaluative techniques have led to various beliefs and expectations about various types of technology. This chapter is primarily concerned with providing a general introduction to the use of technology as a means of examining work practices and enhancing communication within health settings and in particular in the A and E department.

Information within the chapter aims to explain some of the misconceptions surrounding the terms 'technology' and 'information technology' and discusses the application of technology within A and E nursing. Information also sets the scene for further discussion and debate within the reader's own area of clinical practice. Points for discussion within the chapter, in the form of questions, are designed to help the reader consider in detail various areas of the chapter and should provide a basis upon which the reader can develop themes and issues further.

As with all chapters within the book the reader may not agree with ideas and perceptions put forward. Other readers may feel that important points have been missed or omitted. Unfortunately this chapter cannot cover all issues of concern to readers. To overcome this the chapter is organized in sections that can be dipped into and read in conjunction with other texts. Alternatively the chapter provides a wealth of ideas if read from cover to cover.

References at the end of the chapter should also help readers to develop further ideas and information presented within the text.

DEFINITIONS

Searching through the literature produces many and varied examples of the use and effect of technology in health care. Similarly, articles generally detail information technology applications. While technology and information technology are described, few attempts are made to define these terms.

The Concise Oxford English Dictionary (1987) defines technology as 'the science of practical or industrial art' and offers the definition of information as 'desired items of knowledge'.

BACKGROUND TO INFORMATION TECHNOLOGY IN HEALTH CARE

In the 1950s health care information systems were used mainly to store information on large mainframe computers (Alexander, 1992). Defects in these early systems became apparent over the years. In 1979, the Royal Commission on the National Health Service pointed to defects in the arrangements for amassing statistics and said that there should be a forum for considering information matters (Connah and Lancaster, 1989). It was widely agreed that much of the information was of a poor quality and was in a form unsuitable for day-to-day use by operational staff.

This was the background to the setting up, in 1980, of the Steering Group on Health Services Information, chaired by Edith Korner. Alexander (1992) writes that the recommendations of this committee have been 'catalysts in the evolution of health care information systems'. Identifying what information is stored and in what form it is stored led to the term MBDS – Minimum Basic Data Set. The ICD-9 (International Classification of Disease) codes (Arbour, 1978), a set of clinical codings for disease conditions, now complement the Minimum Basic Data Set. As health care providers begin to realize the benefits of information technology, more demands are being placed on the system designers. Health care professionals are no longer satisfied with systems which purely collect and store basic clinical data. Linking health care activities to cost is currently high on the budget holders' agenda in health authorities and trusts. Diagnostic related groups (DRGs) (Fetter, 1988) are now commonplace in the resource management of health care, as are nursing management information systems or ward management information systems.

HEALTH CARE TECHNOLOGY

The subject of technology in health care often involves discussion about machinery or equipment. Information technology, however, tends to be seen as computers. These popular misconceptions often result in a blinkered approach towards any topic concerning technology or information technology. Stocking (1992) argues for an internationally accepted definition of medical technology covering the whole of medical practice: the drugs, equipment and procedures used in medical care, singly or in combination, and the infrastructure for their use. Stocking questions the decision making process for purchase of medical technology, writing that 'a whole range of factors and people influence the introduction and use of medical technology'. Health care technology is perhaps a more favourable term as this more aptly describes the equipment and procedures used in health care, singly or in combination, and the infrastructure for its use. Nursing is perhaps the single largest input to patient care, with a large proportion of a hospital's resources spent on nursing staff. It is, however, doctors and not nurses who have historically been central to any decision making process regarding purchasing of technology. Nurses have had to be content with mentioning to the doctors how advantageous certain items of technology would be if they could be purchased. Political pressure and human behaviour can of course influence choice of purchase as too can local and national management initiatives and sales promotion by the industries concerned. Stocking (1992) argues that all countries need a system for technology assessment and dissemination of that information.

Points for discussion

● How would you define technology in A and E?

● What reasons are given for the purchase of technology in your A and E department?

● How does your A and E department adopt a team approach to the purchase and introduction of new health care technology?

● How well is the technology assessed and evaluated before it is purchased?

Stocking (1992) cites Rogers' (1983) five characteristics of innovation. These can be useful when health care technology is assessed:

relative advantage, compatibility, complexity, observability and trialability (whether they can be tested out).

It is important that health care professionals are able to make some distinctions between technology and information technology. This chapter continues by explaining these differences in more detail.

INFORMATION TECHNOLOGY

The *NHS Handbook* (Connah and Lancaster, 1989) states that:

> information is fundamental to all aspects of health care provision. It is essential in enabling clinical care of individual patients, it is the basis of both operational and strategic management and it underlies the measurement and monitoring of public health.

Huczinski and Buchanan (1991) define information technology as the term used for all types of computer hardware and software, office equipment and telecommunications. Stewart (1986) defines information technology as a general term for computers and other methods of handling information electronically. It is these 'other methods' that tend to be disregarded in the literature. It can be argued that most health care providers see information technology as computers and computer systems. Alexander (1992) writes that most of us know computers can store information but it is the complex way of collecting and expressing that information to the users that generously enhances the role of information technology in health care.

Huczinski and Buchanan (1991) state that information technology is characterized by a fundamental duality that has not yet been fully realized. This duality is seen, on the one hand, in technology that can be applied to automated operations, replacing the human body with a technology allowing for continuity and control of processes and on the other hand that same technology simultaneously generates information about the underlying productive and administrative processes through which an organization accomplishes its work. At present, information technology in British health care is developing its information generation about the underlying productive and administrative processes but has a great distance to travel if it is to achieve applied technology for automated processes directly affecting patient care.

Information technology systems can be implemented from both a top-down or bottom-up approach (Bloomfield, 1992) and evidence is available in support of both methods. It is argued that a top-down approach ensures that only essential information is captured and resources are not wasted collecting irrelevant data. However, McDonnell and Jones (1991) state that information technology systems are only as good as the people who use them. Data will be relevant and accurate only if those people who input the information understand why they are collecting it, its purpose and how it will enhance patient care. For information technology to be effective it needs to be seen as a sophisticated tool to assist A and E staff.

The impact of information technology on health care depends on the understanding by the systems designers of the needs of the users and the users' understanding of the possibilities and constraints of the systems.

Points for discussion

- Consider the staff inputting the information onto computer systems in your A and E department. Why are they collecting the information? What is its purpose and how will it enhance patient care?

- What answers would the input staff give to these questions?

- Who are the designers of the information technology systems used in or by your A and E department?

- If you evaluate the information technology systems which affect your A and E department, how responsive to the department's needs and requirements do you consider the system designers have been?

RESOURCE MANAGEMENT DEFINED

Wilson (1992) sees the term 'resource management' as referring to the information needed to control, measure and manage the resources needed and supplied. Wilson identifies four key elements of resource management:

1. improved quality of care;
2. involvement in management by staff;
3. improved information;
4. effective control of resources.

It is the improved information element of resource management which allows health care professionals to review the mix of services and rebalance them within existing resources in their units of control (Wilson, 1992). The NHS Management Executive (1990) defines resource management as 'a complex process with a single aim – to allow total, individual, high quality patient care to be planned, delivered and costed more effectively.'

Information technology systems can generate this information element which we have previously been unable to capture. From a wider perspective, the role of information technology within the context of resource management can be seen as a tool to provide health care professionals with the necessary information to allow them to make informed decisions, review the mix of services and improve the quality of care while having effective control of the available resources.

NURSE MANAGEMENT INFORMATION SYSTEMS

McDonnell and Jones (1991) write that 'systems of information technology are less important in themselves than the way in which that information is disseminated'. System design and its relevance to the user must also be considered if we are to discuss the role of information technology systems in nursing. If the most important feature of information technology is the information dissemination and the main provider and disseminator of that information is the nurse then a nursing management information system interlinked with other computer systems must be the most effective way to apply information technology in the hospital health care setting.

Wilson (1992) writes that one of the key issues in implementing resource management is to have a nurse management information system which will 'cover all nursing requirements but is as simple as possible for staff to use it to its full advantage'. Wilson describes the elements of any nurse management information system as having three main components:

1. a workload measure;
2. rostering of staff by grade and skill mix to give a good quality of care;
3. care planning as a mechanism to record, monitor and audit the level and quality of care.

Harrow (1988) states that the introduction of computer based information systems into the wards will allow nurses to become totally responsible for the use of their resources and to be able to make precise informed decisions on patient care by providing adequate and accurate data. The role of information technology in health care can again be seen as a sophisticated tool providing nurses with the information to enable improvement in services to patients, to plan and to enhance the quality of care. This information can enable a more efficient use of resources – 'the ultimate beneficiary being the patient' (Harrow, 1988). Baird (1992) argues that better information has a price that must be balanced against improved quality and efficiency in health care planning and provision.

Points for discussion

- What nurse or ward management information systems have been installed in your hospital setting?

- What design features have been included to meet the A and E department's needs and requirements?

- If a system has not as yet been installed, what features would you consider important to meet the A and E department's needs and requirements?

- Is the senior nurse of the A and E department able to feel totally responsible for the use of A and E resources?

- Can the senior nurse make precise, informed decisions on patient care issues and provide adequate and accurate data to support those decisions?

INTEGRATED SYSTEMS

The *NHS Handbook* (Connah and Lancaster, 1989) gives details of the 38 targets for the WHO European Region. Target 35 states that 'Before 1990, member states should have health information systems capable of supporting their national strategies for Health For All'.

While the NHS is moving towards integrated health information systems there is no documentation to suggest that this approach has been adopted nationally. System integration in the United Kingdom appears to be largely piecemeal and fragmented, each hospital deciding its own information technology requirements and introducing systems to meet those requirements. Geiger (1988) writes that even at many of those hospitals with relatively comprehensive support from information technology, integration is missing. Geiger (1988) leads us into an interesting scenario of total systems integration allowing a vision of comprehensive information technology support for the nursing sister at ward level. Geiger states that 'systems integration must be balanced with the benefits it will accrue' and that 'there is little benefit in providing ward sisters with information on expenditure if they do not have a budget within which to work'.

There is little benefit in providing information on nursing requirements based upon patient dependency if there is no forum within which staffing requirements can be discussed, addressed and resolved. Hoy (1987) discusses the great wealth of knowledge, information and experience which has been accumulated in the application of the computer in all aspects of health care. He sees differing groups doing the same thing, not cooperating or contacting each other, causing fragmentation of effort. Case mix systems aim to reduce this fragmentation of effort and duplication of information by aggregating patient data. Information technology's role in this context can be seen as acting as a sophisticated tool used by differing groups of health care providers. The advances in information technology now make full system integration possible. Hoy (1988) stresses the need for an integrated and cooperative effort. Baird (1992) cautions that the organization must be mature enough to act on the superior management information it receives and so be prepared to change behaviour as a consequence. If this does not happen then much of the benefit of integrated case mix systems will be lost and case mix may become an expensive way of producing discharge summaries.

Points for discussion

- What are the information requirements of your A and E department?

- How is this information currently collected?

- Is the same information collected more than once – for example, patient's name, age and initial diagnosis?

- How could the system of information collection be improved?

COMPUTER TECHNOLOGY – APPLICATIONS IN NURSING

Watt (1987) writes that nursing, like any other profession, requires constantly to examine the use of computers in its organization; nurses must turn to computer technology to assist them in recording accurate and up-to-date information. Watt sees information technology's role in nursing primarily as 'allowing nurses to nurse. Freeing nurses from the complex and time consuming task of manually documenting information about staff and patients'. Litchfield (1992) argues that it is no longer adequate to express the benefits of computer technology in terms of saving time, freeing nurses or bringing nurses in line with other health care professionals: 'It is the impact on the nature of nursing that is important'.

While there is a vast difference between the views of the two authors on the benefits and use of information technology in nursing, it could be argued that in order to evaluate the impact of information technology on nursing, nurses must first have experienced the benefits of using it in their profession; for example, computerized care planning (Standley, 1992), computerized nursing workload and dependency data (Wilson, 1992) and computer assisted learning packages (CAL)

(McCormac and Jones, 1992). Hoy (1988) describes nursing as a caring concept and therefore very difficult to define. In addition to this he says nurses also coordinate the work of other health care professionals for the patient's benefit and sees there being complete sharing of information between professionals with the nurse as the central hub accepting a high profile role supported by immediate access to information.

Kelly (1991) describes how computer training packages are available for staff to help them develop confidence in and awareness of computer technology. Five out of nine of the packages are designed specifically for nurses. Basford (1991) reviews a computer software package about coping with stress, stating that it has endless applications within the health care professions. The above issues demonstrate the diversity of computer technology for health care professionals and nurses in particular. No longer is the computer seen as just an administrative tool for clerical staff to register patient details. In addition to this, a wide range of software packages is now available for patients to use. Nelson-Smith (1991) describes how computers can be a welcome distraction and novelty and lists many real benefits of computers for children in hospital. Computer programmes are available for children from age two upwards.

Points for discussion

● How is staff rostering managed in the A and E department?

● If a manual system is used, what grade of staff manage it?

● What are the cost implications of managing staff rostering manually?

● What are the cost implications of using a computer system to manage staff rostering?

FUTURE APPLICATIONS FOR INFORMATION TECHNOLOGY IN HEALTH CARE

Hoy (1988) describes two main areas for future development:

1. Single record for each patient held in a common database, to which all health care related systems have access. This record could be a comprehensive health record including community or primary care as well as hospital care data.
2. Linked networks is the second area of future development, with standardization of data administration, usage and definition.

Huczinski and Buchanan (1991) cite Marien (1989) who identifies 125 actual or potential impacts of information technology. Under the heading of health and health care are:

- computer assisted diagnosis and cost analysis;
- smart card health and medical history recording;
- computer as home health advisor;
- computerphobia and technostress.

Alexander (1992) provides us with a vision of the resource managed hospital in the 21st century – a hospital information system which will monitor the costs of every activity from laundry to surgery. However, it can be argued that the cost of every activity is not nearly as important an issue as the value of every activity or the benefit gained by the activity.

Some of the above mentioned future developments are being realized in 1994. Several research projects are currently being undertaken throughout the United Kingdom to examine the feasibility of integrated single care records. Several general practitioner practices have tested computer assisted diagnostic tools. Cross (1992) describes details of the Hammersmith and Queen Charlotte Special Health Authority in West London who have ordered computers worth £2.2 million to support its move towards 'electronic X-ray images making X-rays on film a thing of the past'. If we reconsider Huczinski and Buchanan's description of information technology as being characterized by fundamental duality then the organization is the hospital and its work is the coordinated delivery of efficient and effective high quality patient care. As discussed previously, information technology in health care is gradually developing its information generating strategies.

While computer usage in clinical practice is increasing, again the information technology is used as a tool to aid the health care professional and not as a replacement for the health care professional. The role of information technology can be as diverse or as specific as the health care provider requires. Watt (1987) states that computers 'are only a tool to help them (nurses) and they must understand the capabilities as well as the limitations of the technology'. In agreement, Wilson (1992) writes that computer systems are 'there to help (nurses) ... but will never replace them and their professional judgement'.

Points for discussion

- How many activities within the A and E department could be performed by a sophisticated computerized system?
- Is replacing the human body with a technology that allows for control of processes a realistic scenario for future consideration?

In other words, can surgeons be replaced by computer technology which controls and performs surgical operations or clinical investigations on patients?

● How could a computer be used to benefit patients in the A and E setting?

COMPUTER TECHNOLOGY – ACCIDENT AND EMERGENCY APPLICATIONS

Bradley (1992) asks if total computerization of the emergency setting will eventually become reality. The United Kingdom should be aware of the developments in the United States as it often follows that what happens in the United States today will be transferred to the United Kingdom tomorrow.

Bradley describes eight areas of A and E work where computer systems have become a reality in the United States, including:

1. paramedic notes relayed to the receiving hospital for information;
2. computer assisted triage where the triage nurse is given preset standard questions following input of patient's age and chief presenting complaint;
3. a system whereby the names and problems of patients in the waiting area are visible to the nurse in charge;
4. patient location monitors providing information such as room number, name, chief complaint and laboratory results plus assigned nurse and doctor plus accompanying information regarding relatives or bed status for admission;
5. bedside computers which interface and communicate with other machines. These can be for intravenous pumps, cardiac monitors, pulseoximeters and laboratory results;
6. medication retrieval from computerized pharmacy machines with inbuilt calculations for child dosages.

Bradley continues by discussing computerized discharge instructions for patients, which will be discussed in more detail later, and also explains that an endless array of reports will be available for quality improvement, reinforcing the fact that whatever information is entered into the computer, a report can come out of it.

UK A and E departments are using varying levels of computer technology. Government legislation specifies the minimum information required from patient registration systems in the A and E department and many departments have systems which are only able to provide this minimum information.

In consideration of the potential applications of computer technology in A and E, this chapter will now continue by examining the practical application of computer technology in one A and E department.

COMPUTER TECHNOLOGY – PRACTICAL APPLICATION IN ONE A AND E DEPARTMENT

Checkout© is a computerized information software package providing personal individualized discharge instructions for patients being cared for in A and E settings. Through using relatively simple keyboard commands and a user-friendly Windows screen, medical and nursing staff can compile comprehensive aftercare instructions for their patients. Those instructions relate to any illness or injury the patient has presented with and also gives details of treatment, medications and follow-up care prescribed for the patient. The language used is clear and concise and easily understood by most patients attending. The system is used in approximately 100 hospital A and E departments in the United States and is currently used in several departments in the United Kingdom.

The North Staffordshire Royal Infirmary A and E department implemented the system in 1990 following 12 months of planning and discussion coordinated by two members of nursing staff. Previously discharge information available to the patients had taken the form of preprinted sheets containing general information or verbal advice given by the health professionals.

A multidisciplinary group worked within an action plan in order to implement and evaluate the system. The group consisted of a general practitioner, health visitor and district nurse liaison officer, A and E clinical nurse specialist, senior pharmacist, consultant paediatrician, resource management project officer, physiotherapist, A and E consultant and medical and nursing staff from the A and E department.

The Checkout© text was altered and tailored to ensure relevance and benefit for patients in the A and E department. The text was then face and content validated by a consultant paediatrician, A and E consultant and senior pharmacist. An intensive training programme was arranged for all the A and E staff. For demonstration, training and practice, the computer system was initially set up in an office allowing easy access for the staff at any time and ensuring a degree of privacy for those who felt apprehensive about computers. The system was fully introduced into the department on 3 December 1990. Approximately 100–130 patients received individualized instructions per 24-hour period. The system was introduced for the patients' benefit and describes their diagnoses and prescribes the medications all in

for Janet Dutton, Friday, February 15, 1991, 2:17 am

IMPORTANT: We have examined and treated you today on an emergency basis only. This is not a substitute for, or an effort to provide, complete medical care. Tell your own doctor about any new or lasting problems. It is impossible to recognize and treat all injuries or illnesses in a single Accident unit visit. If you had X-rays taken, we will review them again within 24 hours. We will call you if there are any new suggestions. After leaving, you should **FOLLOW THE INSTRUCTIONS BELOW.**

You were treated today by Dr J Nash. Your discharging nurse was I Wood.

LIGAMENT SPRAIN
You have sprained your **left ankle** ligament(s). Ligaments are ropelike bands that hold bones to each other. You have stretched and torn some of your ligament fibres. If you can keep swelling down, you will feel better sooner. Three things help to keep swelling down in the first 48 hrs:

1. Elevation is most important. Keep the injured part above the level of your heart if you can.
2. Ice packs are very helpful. Use a piece of cloth between the ice pack and the injured part to prevent frostbite.
3. Strapping is helpful for arms and legs when you must be up and around.

CONSULT YOUR DOCTOR if you have worsening pain or swelling. However, discomfort can continue for several **MONTHS** following this injury.

TUBIGRIP
This elastic bandage helps support an injured part. It helps protect the limb or joint and also helps to keep swelling down.

Make sure the Tubigrip does not roll down to form a band around the injured limb. This band could stop the flow of blood through the limb. Take the Tubigrip off when you go to bed and put it back on before getting up. If you get any colour change, numbness or increased swelling of the limb, remove the Tubigrip, raise the injured limb and **CONTACT THE ACCIDENT AND EMERGENCY DEPARTMENT OR YOUR FAMILY DOCTOR for advice.**

IBUPROFEN (Brufen, Nurofen).
This medicine is an effective anti-inflammatory medicine. It can also relieve pain. Most people will not have any side effects. Some will develop a stomach ache when taking the tablets.

A rare side effect is allergy. This would show up as shortness of breath or wheezing, rash or itching. If you have any allergy symptoms, or any new or severe symptoms, **CONSULT A DOCTOR.**

To avoid stomach ache, take each dose with solid food. Dose: 200 or 400 mg 3 times a day.

THESE ARE YOUR FOLLOW-UP INSTRUCTIONS!

If you are not better in ten days, contact Dr Smith

Contact him/her sooner if you become worse. **You can reach Dr Smith**

Tel:
AS ALWAYS, YOU ARE THE MOST IMPORTANT FACTOR IN YOUR RECOVERY. Please follow the instructions above carefully. Take your medicines as prescribed. Most important, see a doctor again as discussed. If you have problems that we have not discussed, **CALL OR VISIT YOUR DOCTOR.** If you can't reach your doctor, return to the Accident unit.

*I understand the instructions, written above, and discussed in the Accident unit.

....
Patient or responsible person

....
Doctor or qualified nurse

CIGARETTE SMOKING
Smoking is a major health problem! The facts are clear that cigarette smoking will shorten your life. It will cause a great deal of illness along the way. If you need help stopping, talk to your family doctor.

SEATBELTS
There is no doubt that seatbelts save lives in both front and back seats. Every day in the Accident unit we see how people without seatbelts are more severely hurt. We always buckle up. Please do the same!

These instructions were prepared and printed in 60 seconds

Figure 6.1 Aftercare instructions (reprinted by kind permission of the *British Journal of Nursing*).

lay terms. It allows patients to make informed decisions about their after-care and considerably enhances the quality and standard of discharge information available to the A and E patient.

An example of a discharge instruction is shown in Fig. 6.1.

More sophisticated systems are now being applied to A and E departments, heavily packaged and marketed as all-singing, all-dancing systems. However, departments should proceed with caution and heed Bradley's comments (1992), noting that 'Computers will not solve all of our problems, in fact they will probably create new dilemmas'. A and E staff need to ensure that the systems are designed primarily for their benefit and that the designers understand and listen to their needs.

Computerized poisons information is now available in many A and E departments and provides a valuable resource for patient care. Again, A and E staff must ensure they are adequately informed regarding the benefits of introducing such a system before a decision to purchase is made. UK computer software is also available (QA Software, 1992), to assist with *Accident and Emergency Monitor* nursing quality audit (Dutton *et al.*, 1991) and *Criteria For Care* demand modelling and dependency system for A and E nursing workload estimate (North Lincolnshire Health, 1991).

Saunders *et al.* (1989) describe the development of a computer simulation model of emergency department operations. There are 'multiple levels of preemptive patient priorities'. Each patient is assigned an individual nurse and doctor and all the standard tests, procedures and consultations are incorporated. The authors describe how all these patient service processes are allowed to proceed simultaneously, sequentially, repetitively or through a combination of these. The variables are altered through simulation and effects on patient throughput time, queue size and rates of resource utilization are monitored. The authors describe this as 'a potentially useful tool that can help predict the results of changes in the emergency department system without actually altering it'.

Points for discussion

- How can a computer system improve communication in the A and E setting?

- What would you want from a computer system in A and E?

- How could a computer assist the triage nurse?

- How can we measure the effect of new technology in the A and E department?

- How much involvement should nursing staff have in the selection and development of new technology?

CONCLUSION

Bradley (1992) sees computers offering nursing a future where more time is spent delivering care instead of documenting it and also providing nurses with the ammunition to make great strides in their search for excellence in emergency practice.

Health care technology of whatever form is not a fad which will eventually become unpopular. It is here to stay and every health care professional should be aware of this. A positive attitude can be adopted, viewing technological advances as of benefit to staff and patients alike, or an apathetic, intolerant attitude can be adopted which may ultimately result in loss of control in the decision making process. For nursing to benefit from technology there should be some control in its selection, purchase and implementation. This sophisticated tool may be used by A and E nurses to their advantage or ignored at their peril.

REFERENCES

Alexander, M. (1992) *Information Technology – A Student Learning Package*, Leeds Polytechnic Publication, Leeds.

Arbour, A. (1978) *International Classification of Diseases*, 9th edn, Commission on Professional and Hospital Activities (CPHA).

Baird, R. (1992) Running out of steam. *Health Service Journal*, **102**(5306), 26–7.

Basford, P. (1991) Software review – coping with stress. *Nursing Times*, **87**(42), 57.

Bloomfield, B. (1992) Top down, botton up. *Health Service Journal*, **102**(5288), 20–2.

Bradley, V. (1992) President's message. Computer systems: answers to your prayers. *Journal of Emergency Nursing*, **18**(3), 181–2.

Concise Oxford English Dictionary (1987) 7th edition, Oxford University Press, Oxford.

Connah, B. and Lancaster, S. (1989) *NHS Handbook*, 4th edn, National Association of Health Authorities/Macmillan Press Ltd, London.

Cross, M. (1992) *Golden Age of Films to History*. *Health Service Journal*, **102**(5300), 37.

Dutton, J.M., Grylls, S.L. and Goldstone, L.A. (1991) *Accident and Emergency Monitor. An Audit of the Quality of Nursing Care in Hospital Accident and Emergency Departments*, Gale Centre Publications, Loughton, Essex.

Fetter, R. (1988) Information systems requirements, in *Case Mix Management by Organisation. Towards New Hospital Information Systems*, (eds A.E. Bakker, J.R. Schenner and J.L. Williams), Elsevier, Amsterdam.

Geiger, P. (1988) *Integrating For Effect*. Proceedings of European Conference on Nursing – The Impact of Information Technology, Leeds Polytechnic, pp. 56–62.

Harrow, M.A. (1988) *The Nursing Perspective on Resource Management*. Proceedings of European Conference on Nursing – The Impact of Information Technology, Leeds Polytechnic, pp. 67–71.

Hoy, R. (1987) Computers and nursing: a scenario, in *Computers and Their Applications in Nursing*, (ed. R. Hoy), J.B. Lippincott, Philadelphia, pp. 72–86.

Hoy, R. (1988) *"Quo Vadis"*; from Nursing – The impact of information technology (conference paper) pp. 2–10.

Huczinski, A. and Buchanan, D. (1991) Advanced technology and work organisation, in *Organisational Behaviour: An Introductory Text*, 2nd edn, (eds A. Huczinski and D. Buchanan), Prentice Hall International (UK) Ltd, Hemel Hempstead, pp. 325–63.

Kelly, J. (1991) High-tech teach-in. *Nursing Times*, 87(48), 59–60.

Litchfield,M. (1992) Computers and the form of nursing to come. *International Journal of Health Informatics*, 1, 7–10.

Marien, M. (1989) IT: you ain't seen nothing yet, in *Computers in Human Context*, (ed. T. Forrester), Basil Blackwell, Oxford, pp. 41–7.

McCormac, K. and Jones, B.T. (1992) A lesson in reality. Computing in practice; information management and technology. *Nursing Times*, 88(14), 55–7.

McDonnell, U. and Jones, A. (1991) Human resources. *Nursing Times*, 87(51), 42–3.

Nelson-Smith, J. (1991) Programs for play. *Nursing Times*, 87(42), 55–7.

NHS Management Executive (1990) *What is Resource Management?* Department of Health, Resource Management Unit, London.

North Lincolnshire Health (1991) *Criteria For Care. Demand Modelling and Dependencies In Accident and Emergency Departments* (unpublished).

QA Software and Consultancy (1992) *Accident and Emergency Monitor*. Computerised Data Analysis, QA Software, Lincoln.

Rogers, E. (1983) *Diffusion of Innovations*, 3rd edn, Free Press, New York.

Saunders, C.E. Makens, P.K. and Leblanc, L.J. (1989) Modelling emergency department operations using advanced computer simulation systems. *Archives of Emergency Medicine*, 18(2), 134–7, 140–3.

Standley, M. (1992) Systems of care. Computing in practice: information management and technology. *Nursing Times*, 88(6), 53–5.

Stewart, R. (1986) The manager and change, in *The Reality of Management*, 2nd edn, (ed. R. Stewart), Pan Business Management, London, pp. 165–85.

Stocking, B. (1992) The future starts here. *Health Service Journal*, 102(5322), 26–8.

Watt, S. (1987) Applications of computers in nurse management, in *Computers and Their Applications in Nursing*, (ed. R. Hoy), J.B. Lippincott, Philadelphia, pp. 1–16.

Wilson, J. (1992) Data systems can boost nursing care. Resource management. *Professional Nurse*, 7(5), 325–8.

CHAPTER 7

Solving problems in the A and E department: a basis for nursing practice

L. Sbaih

INTRODUCTION

Nursing is undergoing many changes particularly in relation to the application of theory to practice and the use of problem solving strategies within the clinical environment. The purpose of this chapter is to examine some of these issues and the reader is expected to consider the value of all points put forward within their own area of clinical practice.

The organization of the chapter is such that a wide range of ideas has been introduced. Within the chapter ideas have been adapted to A and E and it is up to the reader to consider which areas of the chapter may be viable in practice and to confirm this by putting such ideas into practice and evaluating them.

One of the themes of the book is thinking and doing and this is explicitly addressed within this chapter. One of the themes of the chapter is evaluation of the relationship of theory to practice and the need for nurses to consider and then accept or reject information based upon reliable evidence formulated by those expected to use theory to enhance practice.

The chapter has been designed as one that can be dipped into and the various sections provide information that can be read in isolation, although browsing through the whole chapter will give a clearer impression of the framework suggested for solving problems and how it relates to other parts of the chapter. References at the end of the chapter are viewed as a introduction to other information available on the relationship of theory to practice and the reader is invited to pursue the debate further through the literature presented in this list.

PROBLEM SOLVING IN A AND E

Hurst *et al.* (1991) consider problem solving to be:

> ... one of the most important changes in nursing during the last decade

> (p. 1444)

and the application of problem solving strategies in nursing has resulted in a move from a disease orientated approach to what may be considered holistic and individualized nursing (Henderson, 1982; Aggleton and Chalmers, 1986; Hurst *et al.*, 1991).

Points for discussion

- How many problem solving strategies have been applied in your A and E department?
- Outline the advantages relating to the use of care related problem solving strategies within your department.
- Outline the disadvantages relating to the use of care related problem solving strategies within your department.

Nursing has still to develop suitable problem solving strategies (Walsh and Ford, 1989; Hurst *et al.*, 1991). Where strategies do exist nurses continue to rely on experience and a belief in what has worked before rather than using reflective practice (Walsh and Ford, 1989). Such an approach potentially reduces the individualization of care delivery and may not take into account such issues as communication and consideration of the views held by those involved in care giving and receiving (Benner, 1984). Benner continues by stating that expert nurses may view the patient and immediate environment holistically. However, knowledge and practice are intertwined and 'difficult to articulate' (Meerabeau, 1992, p. 108).

Having difficulty in articulating knowledge and its relationship to practice may also suggest a need for the nurse to consider that practice and its effect upon those involved in the care giving and receiving process if holistic, individualized care is to be recognized and achieved to the satisfaction of all involved.

Points for discussion

- Do problem solving strategies require development within your department?
- How may such development take place?

THEORIES OF PROBLEM SOLVING

Hurst *et al.* (1991) cite work by Newell and Simon (1972) and Chi and Glaser (1984) and introduce two theories of problem solving. The first theory divides problem solving into two specific thinking activities:

1. the process of understanding;
2. the solving phase.

Problem solving, to be successful, requires the individual to:

1. understand the problem;
2. apply strategies for solving the problem.

It should also be noted that moving through the stage of understanding towards the stage of solving may increase the number of recognized problems and issues (Hurst *et al.*, 1991).

With reference to this particular theory of problem solving the type of perceived problem should be recognized as either administrative or care related.

Administrative: Writing the departmental off duty may be placed comfortably within this theory of problem solving.

Care related: Other issues such as recognition of the severity of the patient's pain may be harder to establish within such a theory.

Example 1 Writing the off duty

1. Information
   - 15 nurses in the A and E department
   - 2 wish to have weekend 1 off
   - 6 wish to have weekend 2 off
   - no one wishes to have weekend 3 off
   - 4 wish to have weekend 4 off

2. Understand the problem
   - Unbalanced number of requests to meet the needs of the department skill mix

3. Apply strategies for solving the problem
   - 4 nurses required for the early shift
   - 4 nurses required for the late shift
   - 4 nurses required for the night shift
   - Negotiation required to match needs of the department to needs of the nursing staff

4. Any other problems?
   - Yes, not enough nurses to cover weekend 2 even if all nurses work

Example 2 The patient in pain

1. Information
   - Patient has just arrived in A and E and is complaining of pain in his right foot

2. Understand the problem
   - The patient is in pain in his right foot

3. Apply strategies for solving the problem
   - Non-invasive techniques – reposition foot, keep warm
   - Invasive techniques – analgesia

4. Any other problems?
   - Has the patient described the pain adequately?
   - Has the patient any allergies?
   - Have any strategies been tried prior to the patient's arrival in A and E?

Pain is subjective (McCaffery, 1979) and therefore open to interpretation by those involved in the process of assessment, care giving and receiving. It may be difficult for the patient to describe their pain and for the nurse to understand what is being stated about the patient's pain (Whitis, 1985).

Point for discussion

● How may this theory of problem solving be employed in your A and E department?

Another theory of problem solving is the stages model theory (Hill, 1979). This particular theory of problem solving can be broken down into stages and may be closely associated with the nursing process (Hurst *et al.*, 1991):

Stage 1 Problem identification;
Stage 2 Problem assessment. Problems are identified and broken down into various components; other associated problems are recognized;
Stage 3 Planning. Goals are set with regard to prioritization; interventions are selected;
Stage 4 Implementation. The plan is adhered to, practical (doing) and intellectual (thinking) activities are undertaken with due regard to prioritization;
Stage 5 Evaluation. Provides feedback for the whole process and recognition that goals have/have not been achieved, problems have been solved. If problems have not been solved then the process is repeated.

Documentation takes place throughout the whole process.

Adoption of such a problem solving strategy (Hill, 1979) within nursing has resulted in the concept of individualized care (Hurst *et al.*, 1991; Aggleton and Chalmers, 1986; Henderson, 1982) but should be regarded as only one potentially suitable method of problem solving within the A and E department (Robinson, 1992; Stevenson, 1974; Hurst *et al.*, 1991).

As has already been stated a number of authors have raised concerns relating to the concept of individualized care, including concerns about the translation of the nursing process problem solving strategy into clinical practice (Hurst *et al.*, 1991; De la Cuesta, 1983; Walsh and Ford, 1989; Meerabeau, 1992). Hurst *et al.* (1991) highlight the following:

With regard to stage 1 (problem identification):
• Nurses often fail to recognize problems and the relationship of various problems to each other;
• Problems are not always recorded;
• Some problems are dismissed as not important;
• Some problems are oversimplified.

With regard to stage 4 (implementation):
• Nurses may not refer to the plan of care which may be viewed as an academic exercise. This is supported by Hurst *et al.* (1991) and Walsh and Ford (1989).

With regard to stage 5 (evaluation):
• Nurses do not seem to understand this stage; this is reflected in its underuse.

So nurses inadequately recognize problems, implement and evaluate care delivery. Hurst *et al.* (1991) suggest that nurses are comfortable with stage 4 (implementation) as this is viewed as 'doing'. However, 'doing' may take place without reference to prior planning or subsequent evaluation. Planning involves thinking about issues associated with the identified problem and evaluation allows recognition of success or failure to solve problems. All issues require further examination within the clinical area.

Concerns relating to the employment of the nursing process in practice may be due to nurses failing to understand the theory underpinning the process of nursing (Hurst *et al.*, 1991; Walsh and Ford, 1989). In particular, documentation of problem solving associated with the nursing process has raised a number of concerns. According to Walsh and Ford (1989) completion of care plans may be viewed:

... as an academic exercise ... the care given bears little resemblance to the hopes and ideas of those brave enough to change British nursing with this concept.

(p. 141)

Issues relating to the documenting of a problem solving strategy raise further potential problems. Documentation reflects the 'doing' and 'thinking' components of a systematic approach to problem solving but is not a problem solving approach (Walsh and Ford, 1989; Hurst *et al.*, 1991). Solving problems within the clinical area may be reflected within the documentation but occur independently of documentation. However, if documentation has not been completed there may be limited evidence to suggest that a systematic approach has been employed.

Issues raised:

- The nursing process and its associated documentation may be viewed as a valuable method of work organization.
- A and E nurses need to make informed decisions about the use of problem solving strategies within their clinical area.
- Nurses in A and E should reflect the doing and thinking components of any problem solving strategy via documentation.
- Problem solving strategies should reflect the reality of A and E nursing.

Overall the employment of problem solving strategies within the A and E department should include the following:

- They should be adaptable (Hurst *et al.*, 1991; Ali, 1990);
- They should be used to assist in meeting the needs of both the environment and the individual receiving care within the A and E department (Sbaih, 1992b).

The nursing process may be a suitable problem solving approach in A and E but before this can be decided, an investigaiton into what, why, how and when should take place and A and E nurses should pay particular attention to the issues raised by Hurst *et al.* (1991) regarding the application of the various stages of the nursing process within the clinical area.

Points for discussion

- Do you believe the nursing process is a suitable method of problem solving in A and E ?
- What evidence could be used to support your response?

Other issues that also require examination include:

- identification of the role of the nurse in the delivery of continuous care within the A and E environment;
- the position of the nurse within the A and E organization (Hurst *et al.*, 1991; Rafferty and Hardy, 1982; Sbaih, 1992b; Meerabeau, 1992).

Nurses in A and E departments are also required to be aware of and acknowledge the goals of the organization prior to the employment of problem solving strategies. Knowledge of the organization should include an appreciation of the A and E department, organization of the hospital and the National Health Service as all potentially affect the employment of problem solving strategies within the A and E department (Eyre, 1986).

Point for discussion

● How familiar are you with the organizational aims of your A and E department?

The goals of the A and E organization may be closely related to the departmental multidisciplinary philosophy of care and decisions about the organization of care within the A and E environment should be taken with regard to departmental objectives which may include a philosophy of nursing (Hurst *et al.*, 1991; Rafferty and Hardy, 1982; Sbaih, 1992b; Meerabeau, 1992). Both should encourage nurses in A and E to examine issues associated with the provision of care. That is, the 'doing', 'thinking' and organizational elements of care provision should be explored (Sbaih, 1992a) in an area where time is limited (Sbaih, 1992c) and priorities are subject to constant review.

Access to nursing literature may also assist nurses in their exploration of the right method for their particular environment, work load and resources (Hurst *et al.*, 1991) by encouraging discussion and development of thinking which can then be applied to doing nursing in A and E (Kolb, 1984).

Other issues which may also require examination include:

- the development of a philosophy of nursing;
- the development of a multidisciplinary philosophy of care;
- the position of the nurse within the A and E multidisciplinary team;
- the position of the nurse within the hospital organization;
- the use of time in A and E, in particular the relationship of time to care giving and receiving;
- the setting of priorities in A and E and how these may be related to the above points;
- the application of ideas within nursing literature to clinical practice in A and E and how this may encourage reflection and the use of problem solving strategies.

Points for discussion

● Outline the role of the nurse in the delivery of continuous care within the A and E environment.

● What is the position of the nurse within the A and E multidisciplinary team?

THE ORGANIZATION

Mintzberg (1973) identifies three types of organization:

1. Entrepreneurial. This strategy relies upon a leader who makes decisions based upon experience and intuition. As a result of such decision making the organization is able to meet aims and objectives quickly. However, the approach of the leader remains static and is unable to accommodate various interests and views.
2. Adaptive. Decisions often relating to the protection of the organization are taken by a number of people slowly and deliberately, leading to a flexible approach to work.
3. Planning. Decisions are based upon a systematic approach to problem solving and examination of the whole environment. Use of intuition and imagination is encouraged once investigation and analysis has taken place.

Point for discussion

● With reference to Mintzberg's work, how would you view the organization of the A and E department?

THE CRITICAL INCIDENT TECHNIQUE

The critical incident technique (Flanagan, 1954; Crouch, 1991; Whitehead, 1978; Eyre, 1986) and computer assisted problem solving (Hurst *et al.*, 1991) are alternative methods that may be applied to the organization of care. They require further analysis by A and E nurses.

The critical incident technique may be viewed as a technique for considering problems in retrospect and reviewing actions in anticipation of a similar problem being encountered in the future (Eyre, 1986). This is summarized by Whitehead (1978):

> Devise the most economical method of working so that each part of the work is begun at the optimum moment and is ready for use when it is required in the overall plan. This will ensure that the work is approached in the most direct way so that the journey to final completion is as short as possible – made along the critical path.
>
> (p. 114)

According to Whitehead the critical path analysis technique has to be learnt and developed. With specific reference to nursing in A and E the following should be considered in further detail.

Most economical method of working

With the A and E department this can be closely related to the use of time by nurses, patients and their families. Nurses need to consider how time can be shared out to meet the needs of all using the A and E department.

Each part of the work is begun at the optimum moment

Nurses who can recognize how patient needs and associated problems may be dealt with before they occur again are in a better position to provide care when it is most needed.

Ready for use when it is required

Nurses who are familiar with how and when a problem may occur within the A and E department will be in a better position to implement problem solving strategies as and when they are required.

Overall plan

Strategies used to solve problems within the department should fit comfortably into the philosophy of care and overall organizational aims of the department; that is, the overall plan.

Work is approached in the most direct way

Nurses then use methods that have been examined in detail and reapplied to similar situations, problems and issues within the clinical area.

Journey to final completion is as short as possible

This summarizes all the above points – the highest standard of care to the right individual at the right time by the right person.

Critical paths are established via a diagram which is referred to as a 'network' (Whitehead, 1978; Eyre, 1986). The network begins on the lefthand side of the page at a specifically recognized starting point (Sisk and Williams, 1981) and moves to the right where the network finishes (Fig. 7.1).

All events and activities are numbered and arrows indicate the route of the activities as the incident develops. Against the activity is the time taken to complete the activity; for nursing activities, this may be an estimation of the time considered necessary to complete the activity.

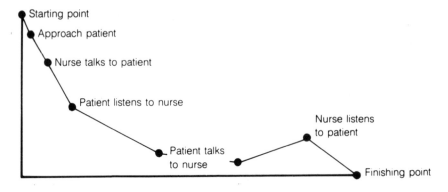

Figure 7.1 The critical path network: talking to a patient in the A and E department

The following critical incident application should also be considered within the A and E department (Crouch, 1991):

1. Information is collected via observation of an incident that is occurring, for example communication between a nurse and patient. Information should be collected by a person who is familar with the action taking place, for example a colleague.

2. Information collected should include the area where the incident took place, what action/s took place, the outcome of the actions and why the action was viewed as effective or not effective (see Example 3 – Talking to a patient).

Colleague observation and the subsequent network should be used at regular intervals as a basis for examination of care delivery and response to patients' verbal and non-verbal requests within the A and E department. According to Crouch, (1991) this process allows '"snapshot" views of the daily work of the nurse' (p. 30) to be gathered. Information gathered can then be used as a basis for discussion about patient care and nurse–patient interaction. Plotting events within a network to create a map of events leading up to the action (Eyre, 1986) may be used as a retrospective exercise allowing for reflection and discussion of the incident and its outcomes. Breaking up an action or series of actions in this way may also assist in the identification of time taken for each component of the action to be completed, therefore providing an indication of the amount of time required to plan patient care within the constraints of the A and E department.

From such discussion particular actions for specific aspects of care can be predicted. Continued analysis of nursing actions in this way can assist in the prediction of problems in care delivery and nurse–patient interaction and should encourage reflection leading to a degree of awareness of the effects of certain approaches to care delivery (Kolb, 1984).

In summary, within the A and E department the critical incident technique approach should include the following:

- Identify the problem.
- Identify the required action.
- Break down the action into stages made up of a number of events and activities.
- Draw the network.
- Examine the network and outline an approach to the action.
- Check the approach against the network.
- Carry out the action with a colleague observing to compare the network against your performance.
- Discuss similarities and update the network accordingly.

Example 3 Talking to a patient

1. Information is collected via observation of an incident that is occurring.

2. Information is collected by a colleague familiar with A and E nursing practices.

3. Information collected includes:
   - the area where the incident took place;
   - observed actions relating to talking and listening, verbal and non-verbal behaviour and body posture of the nurse and patient;
   - the observed outcome of the observed behaviour;
   - actions effective/non-effective.

4. Identify any problems:
   - The nurse spoke to the patient but did not appear to be listening to what the patient had to say.

5. Identify the action that needs to be taken.
   - Further discussion relating to why limited listening by the nurse was observed.
   - The nurse is required to listen to the patient and use non-verbal behaviour to demonstrate active listening to the patient.

6. Break down the action into stages made up of a number of events and activities. This stage may require the support of published literature.
   - The nurse should approach the patient.
   - Introduce herself.

PLEASE NOTE: Information is collected via observation of an incident. Information should be collected by a person familiar with the action taking place ie a colleague.

PART ONE: to be completed by the OBSERVER:

Name _Lynn Sbaih_

Date _14·12·92_

1 Describe the SITUATION observed.

Nurse observed talking to a patient in a cubicle. Patient talking to nurse but difficult to establish if nurse listening to the patient.

2 The situation should now be broken down into a series of EVENTS/ACTIVITIES. These should be described below and include the persons involved/associated with each event/activity.

1. Nurse approached the patient.
2. Patient looked at the nurse.
3. Nurse spoke to patient - patient listening - patient spoke - nurse's back to patient ?Listening

3 Describe the area where the observed SITUATION took place.

Trolley cubicle A+E

4 For how long did you observe the situation?

Five minutes.

5 Describe the outcome of the SITUATION.

Nurse gave patient information.
Limited information from patient.

6 Were observed actions effective/non-effective? Please give reasons.

Some actions appeared effective - the patient gained information but nurse gained limited information from the patient.

7 Additional comments.

None.

END OF PART ONE: Signature _LL Sbaih_

Time _13 05_

Figure 7.2 Critical incident technique form: talking to a patient.

PART TWO: to be completed by all involved in the situation observed

Names *Lynn Sbaih   Helen Bloggs*

Date *14.12.92*

Taking into consideration information recorded in Part One identify the following.

1 What was the SITUATION observed?

Helen talking to a patient in a trolley cubicle.

2 Indicate any identified problems/issues associated with the SITUATION.

Problem: Helen did not appear to be listening to the patient + limited information obtained from the patient.

3 Identify the ACTION (by nurse/patient/others) that should have been taken within the observed SITUATION (this may be the same as that observed).

Helen talks to patient.
Patient talks to nurse.
Both nurse + patient listen to each other.

4 Break down the ACTION into smaller components/activities/events and identify which should have been undertaken by the nurse, by the patient, by others.

Helen approach patient - introduce herself - sit down next to the patient - eye contact - lean forward towards patient then listen to patient maintaining eye contact + verbal + non-verbal contact.

5 Convert information in 4 into a diagram (network) below:

* Starting point
* Approach patient
* Nurse talks to patient
* Patient listens to nurse   *Nurse listens*
* Patient talks to nurse   ** to patient*
                                      * Finishing point
                                                    *

6 Examine the network and indicate on the diagram the length of time required to complete each event.

7 Examine the network. Does this agree with Part Two, No. 4 (YES)/NO.

Agrees with part two, no. 4

*6. To be discussed further with Helen.

8 Discuss with colleagues and review the approach with reference to the network on the previous page
   Done 14.12.92

9 The action/s should now be evaluated in practice, information should be collected by a person familiar with the action taking place, i.e. a colleague. *To be done 15.12.92*

10 Compare the new action with the network, discuss with colleagues similarities and differences and repeat the process accordingly commencing at stage 1, part 1. *To be done 15.12.92*

11 Additional comments.
   Times for actions to be discussed further with Helen before evaluation in practice can take place - to be reviewed and then to no. 10 tomorrow 15.12.92

END OF PART TWO
Signatures *L. Sbaih*
           H. Bloggs

Time *14.12.92*

- Sit at the patient's height (patient sat in a chair).
- Use verbal communication, talking.
- Use non-verbal communication, posture, leaning forward, nodding head.

7. Draw the network.

8. Examine the network and outline an approach to the action.

9. Check the approach against the network.

10. Carry out the action with a colleague observing to compare the network against your performance.
    - The nurse is required to communicate with a patient and will be observed once again.

11. Discuss similarities and update the network accordingly.

Figure 7.2 gives an example.

Observing a nurse undertaking a number of different actions and breaking these down into their component parts will help determine how much time an action may take and the relationship between time and possible outcomes can then be established.

The critical incident technique and nursing process are both problem solving strategies which may be viewed as similar in their approach to the identification of problems and the search for solutions. Differences are also present and for A and E nurses the one most important difference relates to the use of time (Sbaih, 1992c). The nursing process requires the A and E nurse to solve problems as they are occurring. The critical incident technique allows the A and E nurse to reflect and consider solutions to identified problems within the clinical area. When a similar situation, issue or problem recurs then suitable actions which have resulted from peer review and examination can be applied and re-evaluated. This approach should allow A and E nurses to reflect upon their practice, get to know their environment and explore the use of time and prioritization within the clinical area.

Points for discussion

- Outline how the critical incident technique may be employed within your A and E department.

- What particular incidents would benefit from analysis of actions in this way?

COLLABORATION

Successful examination of the organization of care and its delivery within the A and E department requires the use of collaboration between educators, managers and practitioners (Meerabeau, 1992). This is reflected in the UKCC *Code of Professional Conduct* (1992):

> Work in a collaborative and cooperative manner with health care professionals and others involved in providing care and recognize and respect their particular contributions within the care team.

This is supported by Denyes *et al.* (1989) who view collaboration as a means of analysing the application of nursing theory in clinical practice. They continue their argument by suggesting that integration is a focal issue in the challenge of research, theory and practice in nursing (Denyes *et al.*, 1989; Jennings, 1987; Greenwood, 1984). All those involved in all three areas need to work together to achieve accountability for the profession of nursing as a whole.

However, integration within nursing as a whole is rare (Denyes *et al.*, 1989; Jennings, 1987; Greenwood, 1984) and this has contributed in the past to limited understanding of various parts of the profession, the norm being segregation of research from theory and segregation of theory from practice.

Point for discussion

● How may the use of collaboration assist in the exploration of theory issues in A and E practice?

Denyes *et al.* (1989) suggest that the roles of practitioners and researchers have in the past been isolated from one another. The practitioner has often been required to collect information for the researcher, who has removed him/herself from the clinical area and analyses information for which they are then accredited. Such limited collaboration has led to limited communication, resulting in limited opportunity for evaluation of the process in relation to delivery of patient care by all parties involved. With relation to the UKCC *Code of Professional Conduct* (UKCC, 1992) collaboration is required if all those involved in the delivery of care are to pool their resources of knowledge.

Evaluation has been recognized as an important aspect of a collaborative approach to care (Denyes *et al.*, 1989; Greenwood, 1984; Jennings, 1987) and according to Lancaster (1985), collaboration is dependent upon the following:

1. Contribution
2. Communication
3. Commitment
4. Compatibility
5. Credit

Collaboration between researchers, theorists, educationalists, managers and practitioners is required in A and E. To this may be added the patient and family as they should also be invited to collaborate in the delivery and receipt of their care. Collaboration should be underpinned by communication leading to enhanced commitment and compatibility (Lancaster, 1985). Compatibility between all involved parties must be perceived as positive. Questions, doubts and potential conflict should be addressed by ongoing discussion and feedback. The outcome should be collaboration with credit awarded to all involved in such collaboration.

Example 4 Introducing a new wound dressing technique

A member of staff within the department would like to introduce a new wound dressing technique for a specific A and E client group.

The staff member introduces the idea (contribution), staff from research, education, management, medicine and practice are invited to provide feedback (communication) and put forward their ideas (contribution). Ideas put forward (contribution and commitment) from all involved individuals assist in the development of the original idea. Ideas are checked against the original theme by individuals from all disciplines (compatibility), all staff receive support for ideas put forward (credit), constant feedback is evident (communication).

Point for discussion

● How may the above be employed to establish the process of collaboration within your A and E department?

Collaboration should be viewed as a collection of ideas from a number of perspectives. The more perspectives, the more discussion and the increased possibility of finding solutions to problems, issues and situations occurring within the A and E environment. Collaboration therefore may be a means of identifying suitable problem solving strategies for use within the A and E department.

All collaboration related issues rely upon good verbal and non-verbal communication and an understanding of the process is acknowledged through regular feedback, contribution and evaluation by all group members (Lancaster, 1985). Assumptions about care delivery (Walsh and Ford, 1989) should also be recognized (Denyes *et al.*, 1989) and an understanding of the process is acknowledged through regular feedback and contribution from all group members.

Points for discussion

You may wish to examine the following in relation to a collaborative approach:

- Which nurses should be involved?
- What should be their backgrounds?
- What theoretical preparation of nurses is required?
- How can motivation be maintained?

NURSING THEORY

Points for discussion

- What is a theory?
- How are theorists of nursing used in A and E practice?

According to the *Collins English Dictionary* (1989) theory is defined as a 'system of rules and principles; rules and reasoning, etc. as distinguished from practice'. With reference to this definition, thinking and enquiring is an activity undertaken by most nurses at some time in their professional and private lives (Hardy, 1988). All nurses must at some time consider what they are doing and why; that is, they theorize or speculate, therefore theory has a place in clinical practice. Theorizing involves thinking and considering how things work or are organized (McCaugherty, 1992) and resultant theories are classed as informal and speculative whereas theories associated with rigorous investigation are considered formal and scientific (McCaugherty, 1992). Such theory 'is constructed from the evidence and results of a systematic form of inquiry' (McCaugherty, 1992). The resulting theory may be considered to be accurate and puts forward relationships between various components of a whole (Benner, 1984).

A question asked by Ingram (1991) is related to the purpose of nursing theory. It may be assumed that theory is designed to improve nursing practice (Marriner, 1986). However, there is little evidence to support this assumption (Green, 1985; Webb, 1986; Robinson, 1992; Hardy, 1988; Melia, 1987). According to Ingram (1991), theory may have developed for two main reasons:

1. as a means of professional recognition;
2. as a means of directing the profession via the development of a knowledge base.

Points for discussion

- What is your view of the purpose of theory?
- Are you familiar with any work that has evaluated a theory in practice?

Theory may be viewed in a number of ways by nurses (McCaugherty, 1992; Falco, 1989; Hogan and DeSantis, 1991):

1. as information delivered in the classroom;
2. as frameworks for nursing care, that is, nursing models;
3. as a means of describing nursing;
4. a guide to nursing action;
5. a means of defining the possible outcomes of nursing care;
6. a means of promoting problem solving and thinking about nursing as a whole.

Theory is viewed as being acquired through thinking and reflecting (Kolb, 1984) and is required if practice is to develop and be safe (Benner, 1984).

With reference to all these issues, nursing needs to continue to develop via the process of investigation and then challenge existing knowledge (Walsh and Ford, 1989; Robinson, 1992; Hogan and DeSantis, 1991; Hardy, 1988; Meerabeau, 1992; Denyes *et al.*, 1989; Benner, 1984). Only then can existing theory be evaluated. According to Hardy (1988) and Jolley and Allan (1989) there has been minimal evaluation of theory in practice and this has led to confusion amongst nurses, particularly those working in the clinical area who are expected to translate theory into their everyday work practices.

This is of potential importance as the translation of theory into practice is under increasing examination (Biley, 1991). Many theories of nursing may be considered descriptive, having limited reference to the process of research both during and following their development (Hardy, 1988; Silva, 1986).

Points for discussion

● Should theory be generated within the clinical area or outside the clinical area?

● By whom should theory be generated – the practitioner, the manager, the educator, others?

● Who should evaluated theory in the A and E department?

● At what stage in its development should theory be evaluated?

● What other questions and issues should be considered before more theory is generated?

With reference to the *Collins English Dictionary* (1989) definition, Marquis Bishop (1986) argues that nurses are required to examine the definitions of theory and the process of examination may highlight that there is nothing that can accurately be referred to as nursing theory. She continues by suggesting that nurses should stop trying to find out whether nursing theory does or does not exist.

With reference to clinical practice, Ingram (1991) describes nursing as a 'practice discipline' (p. 350) highly valued by those that practise it (Dyson, 1992). This raises the question of whether nursing requires a theory base, as advocated by many of the theorists (Chinn and Jacobs, 1987; Roper *et al.*, 1983; Orem, 1985).

Alternatively it may be argued that practice in itself requires a basis upon which it can be developed and delivered accurately and safely. For this, theory is required by nurses (Benner, 1984; Marriner, 1986; McCaugherty, 1992).

> Practice without theory is uninformed action and theory without practice is mere 'verbalism'. To lose the value of practice would be to lose the essence of nursing.
>
> *(Dyson, 1992, p. 46)*

Ingram (1991) questions the effects of theory application in practice on manpower and resources. He continues by suggesting that all involved in the generation and inititation of theory in the clinical area should ensure that access can be gained to the contents of the theory by all nurses. Also theory should reflect the reality of nursing in that particular practice area.

Points for discussion

- What is your experience of the translation of theory into the A and E department?
- Was the theory understandable?
- Did it assist you in the development of your nursing role?
- Did it assist in the organization of patient care?
- Did it assist in the delivery of patient care within the A and E department?
- Did it assist in the continuity of care within the A and E department?

Theory may be viewed as a common starting point for all nurses (Chinn and Jacobs, 1987), providing nurses with a common language from which continuity of care can be discussed and developed. The use of theory improves communication for it provides a common language and expression of ideas relating to patient care.

Point for discussion

● If communication is regarded as a problem in the clinical area will a language derived from nursing theory assist nurses in talking to each other, clients and their families in the A and E department?

One important consideration is that nursing theory is made up of values, assumptions and judgements (Ingram, 1991; Benner, 1984; Hardy, 1988) and results in nursing being viewed in various ways (Roper *et al.*, 1983; Orem, 1985). Limited reference to the recognition of values and assumptions has led some theorists to attempt to provide nursing with a single theory (Ingram, 1991). Ingram continues by stating that a single theory has been put forward as a way of attempting to prevent confusion by the use of many theories. Unfortunately, because many nurses may view nursing in many ways (Roper *et al.*, 1983; Orem, 1985; Benner, 1984), a single theory may cause just as much confusion as many theories. Nurses therefore need to be united in their understanding of theory and its potential for development or non-development within the A and E department (Ingram, 1991; Hogan and DeSantis, 1991; Leddy and Pepper, 1985).

Point for discussion

● Which approach applies to A and E nursing, a single theory or a number of theories?

Chinn and Jacobs (1987) believe that theory allows knowledge to develop and suggest that knowledge may be viewed as a power source and used to acquire more power and status for the group of nurses employing and developing theory. With reference to nursing, theory may allow nurses to argue for the need for more knowledge and more resources and ultimately this may lead to more nursing autonomy which in turn may allow more knowledge and autonomy to develop.

Point for discussion

● Discuss this idea with particular reference to the A and E department.

ACQUIRING THE KNOWLEDGE

McCaugherty (1992) cites work by Russell (1967) to illustrate arguments about the acquisition of knowledge. According to Russell, knowledge may be acquired through 'acquaintance', that is, following action, or by 'description', that is, thinking and reference to published work (McCaugherty, 1992).

It may be stated that one method of knowledge acquisition within the clinical area is via 'acquaintance' (Benner, 1984). However, acquisition of knowledge in this way requires the support of reflection (Walsh and Ford, 1989; Benner, 1984; Kolb, 1984).

Alternatively work by Polanyi (1958) uses the terms 'tactic' and 'explicit' to express types of knowledge acquisition. Tactic knowledge is rooted in practice and involves knowledge of issues that cannot be easily placed within words such as feelings and inferences. Such knowledge acquisition may be associated with that gained by 'acquaintance' (Russell, 1967), whilst explicit knowledge is derived from thinking and is expressed via language and is similar to knowledge gained by 'description' (Russell, 1967).

In summary, knowledge may be acquired via the following routes:

1. practice, experience of feelings and inferences – tactic;
2. action – acquaintance;
3. thinking, experience of language – explicit;
4. thought, experience of published work – description.

Point for discussion

● By which method have you acquired your knowledge of A and E nursing?

Nursing knowledge may be rooted in 'tactic' knowledge that is difficult to communicate to others both within and outside the profession (Benner, 1984). Tactic knowledge and knowledge gained through 'acquaintance' both require a degree of educational support and reflection (Benner, 1984; Kolb 1984). McCaugherty (1992) introduces work by Kolb (1984) who uses the term 'double knowledge' in an attempt to explain how knowledge is acquired through doing and thinking. Kolb considers the relationship between doing and thinking to be reflection.

> Kolb argues, knowledge is created through the transformation of experience. Experimentation – trying out ideas and thoughts – serves also to link thinking and doing.
>
> (McCaugherty, 1992, p. 30)

Therefore if the root of a nurse's knowledge is 'tactic' it may still require the addition of 'explicit' knowledge acquired through thinking and reflection for the skill, knowledge and resultant action to develop (Kolb, 1984; Benner, 1984; Walsh and Ford, 1989).

Point for discussion

● How may reflection of practice take place in A and E?

Nursing theory may be regarded as a body of knowledge which should be translated into practice but frequently it is done inadequately for a number of reasons (McCaugherty, 1992; Ingram, 1991; Robinson, 1992). This has resulted in a theory–practice gap (Biley, 1991; McCaugherty, 1991; Cook, 1991). Biley (1991) believes that the nursing process and nursing models have increased the perceived gap between theory and practice whilst others may view the nursing process as popular (Hurst *et al.*, 1991). Biley (1991) views the nursing process and nursing model approach as one that requires thinking; unfortunately nurses have little preparation in styles and approaches to thinking about practice. Traditionally, nursing has grown out of medicine's need to have support (Dingwall *et al.*, 1988) and overall:

> This has required nursing to operate within a set of rules, procedures, policies and rituals that require little or no use of intuitive or analytical thought.
>
> (Biley, 1991, p. 31)

This is supported by Benner (1984) and Walsh and Ford (1989). Robinson (1992) recognizes the need for there to be structure and organization to life and the use of theory may meet this need although not necessarily within the clinical area (Biley, 1991).

With reference to this statement, nursing knowledge cannot be viewed as static for it is constantly developing (Robinson, 1992). Nursing theory and frameworks for care rely upon the assumption that society, health and the environment all form an integral part of nursing (Falso, 1989). These are all constantly developing phenomena and should be reflected in constantly developing nursing knowledge. Current nursing knowledge, therefore, may be viewed as too rigid to allow such action to take place within practice, particularly if nursing is being viewed as primarily a social interaction (Benner, 1984) dependent upon individuals interacting within the environment at any given time.

Robinson (1992) supports work by Stevenson (1974) who suggests that an alternative approach to a 'body of knowledge' should be 'terms of reference'. However, physiological and sociological terms of reference would need to be recognized if the nature of nursing was to be completely encompassed for nursing theory is borrowed from other disciplines such as physiology and psychology (Hogan and DeSantis, 1991; McCaugherty, 1992) and the recognition of the roots of nursing knowledge is required if blending of natural sciences and the social activities of nursing is to take place (Robinson, 1992; Biley, 1991).

In addition, McCaugherty (1992) recognizes that there is a difference between theories of nursing which is new knowledge and theories within nursing which may be considered to be the roots and foundations of nursing knowledge. Unless these concepts are examined in detail nursing cannot develop and move forward (Hogan and DeSantis, 1991; Ingram, 1991).

Point for discussion

● How is theory viewed in A and E?

A theme introduced by Ingram (1991) needing further consideration is that the use of practice without a theory base 'may raise ethical concerns' (p. 353). This is of particular interest in the A and E department where continuity of care is often organized within a short span of time (Sbaih, 1992c). Concerns of an ethical nature may arise and should be addressed by nurses working in A and E. This is supported by Robinson (1992):

> Nursing's uncritical tendency to appropriate the methods and language of what it believes to be a 'science' in an apparent attempt to appear 'scientific' without attempting to consider some of the related philosophical problems is a matter of major concern.
>
> (p. 634)

Point for discussion

● How may this issue be translated into theory use in the A and E department?

According to McCaugherty (1992) theory and practice and the potential gap between them need to be examined in great detail by all nurses. This is supported by Biley (1991) and Cook (1991). With reference to Kolb (1984), 'doing' needs to be followed by a period of reflection and thinking away from the event in order for cause and effect relationships to be fully established and appreciated. This may be difficult for the practitioner in the A and E department. Time for reflection may be unpredictable and is affected by external issues such as tiredness and stress, all of which affect overall motivation.

McCaugherty (1992) believes that nursing theory should be clearly related to nursing practice and that care should be taken as to how much is delivered in the classroom away from the unique person to whom that care is being directed. He states:

> Theoretical descriptions and discussion are an important starting point ... a theoretical springboard into the waters of practice.
>
> (p. 33)

This process should be integrated with the ability, time and permission to stand back and reflect (Kolb, 1984) upon actions taken so that the cause and effect relationship can be accurately developed and

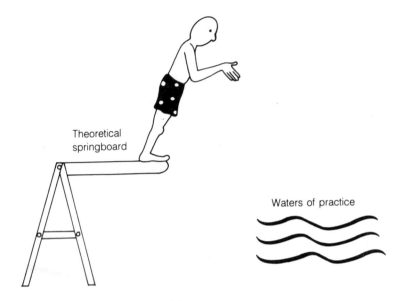

Figure 7.3 The theoretical springboard.

principles considered through thinking applied back to practice (McCaugherty, 1992; Benner, 1984; Biley, 1991).

'Doing' nursing also allows the nurse to learn the hidden rules of skill delivery in the clinical area. Skill practice, if confined to the classroom, cannot be delivered and understood fully (McCaugherty, 1992).

> By watching the master and emulating his efforts ... the apprentice unconsciously picks up the rules of the art including those which are not explicitly known to the master himself.
> *(McCaugherty, 1992, p. 33)*

This watching and copying cannot be done in the classroom; it has to occur in the clinical area and involves putting knowledge into practice and then stepping back and thinking about its relationship to the theory and the effect of its translation into practice. Thus a cause and effect relationship is created that shapes the next similar encounter (Benner, 1984).

ASKING QUESTIONS AND SOLVING PROBLEMS

Hardy (1988) suggests that humour and language that encourages questioning and development are much needed within the nursing theory and problem solving debate. Freedom to consider and examine all theory should be available to all nurses rather than the expectation of conformity to theoretically constructed rules of application.

An imaginative approach is required if more debate of ideas, conflicts and questions is to take place (Hardy, 1988). Finally, but by no means least, Hardy considers the role of the patient to be inadequately addressed within much of the literature with the nurse assuming ideas and roles for the patient rather than finding out what the patient really wants.

Hardy considers that nurses should be clear about the fact that solutions to problems within nursing will not be resolved through the use of theory, but rather by an acknowledgement of different ideas. Also as ideas are generated they should be challenged through ongoing debate and discussion (Hardy, 1988).

Therefore imagination, discussion and an ongoing challenge of various ideas are required if problems are to be recognized and addressed via a knowledge base. Nursing knowledge is required for problem solving in the A and E department but it is not sufficient if other ingredients such as humour, the knowledge of the patient and family, imagination, adaptability, communication and collaboration are missing.

REFERENCES

Aggleton, P. and Chalmers, H. (1986) Nursing research, nursing theory and the nursing process. *Journal of Advanced Nursing,* **11**, 197–202.

Ali, L.C. (1990) Models in accident and emergency. *Nursing Standard,* **5**(3), 33–5.

Benner, P. (1984) *From Novice to Expert: Excellence and Power in Clinical Nursing Practice,* Addison-Wesley Publishing, California.

Biley, F. (1991) The divide between theory and practice. *Nursing,* **4**(29), 30–3.

Chi, M.T.H. and Glaser, R. (1984) Problem solving ability, in *Human Abilities: An Information Processing Approach,* (ed. R.J. Sternberg), Freeman, New York.

Chinn, P.L. and Jacobs, M.K. (1987) *Theory and Nursing: A Systematic Approach,* 2nd edn, C.V. Mosby, St Louis.

Collins English Dictionary (1989) Collins, London.

Cook S.H. (1991) Mind the theory/practice gap in nursing. *Journal of Advanced Nursing,* **16**, 1462–9.

Crouch, S. (1991) Critical incident analysis. *Nursing,* **4**(37), 30–1.

De La Cuesta, C. (1983) The nursing process: from development to implementation. *Journal of Advanced Nursing,* **8**, 365–71.

Denyes, M.J., O'Conner, N.A., Oakley, D. and Ferguson, S. (1989) Integrating nursing theory, practice and research through collaborative research. *Journal of Advanced Nursing,* **14**, 141–5.

Dingwall, R., Rafferty, A.M. and Webster, C. (1988) *An Introduction to the Social History of Nursing,* Routledge, London.

Dyson, J. (1992) The importance of practice. *Nursing Times,* **88**(40), 44–6.

Eyre, E.C. (1986) *Mastering Basic Management,* Macmillan, London.

Falco, S.M. (1989) Major concepts in the development of nursing theory. *Recent Advances in Nursing,* **24**, 1–17.

Flanagan, J.C. (1954) The critical incident technique. *Psychological Bulletin,* **5**, 327–58.

Green, C. (1985) An overview of the value of nursing models in relation to education. *Nurse Education Today,* **5**(6), 267–71.

Greenwood, J. (1984) Nursing research: a position paper. *Journal of Advanced Nursing*, **9**, 77–82.

Hardy, L.K. (1988) Excellence in nursing through debate – the case of nursing theory. *Recent Advances in Nursing*, **21**, 1–13.

Henderson, V. (1982) The nursing process: is the title right? *Journal of Advanced Nursing*, **7**, 103–9.

Hill, C.C. (ed.) (1979) *Problem Solving. Learning and Teaching: An Annotated Bibliography*, Pinter, London.

Hogan, N. and DeSantis, L. (1991) Development of substantive theory in nursing. *Nurse Education Today*, **11**, 167–71.

Hurst, K., Dean, A. and Trickey, S. (1991) The recognition and non-recognition of problem solving stages in nursing practice. *Journal of Advanced Nursing*, **16**, 1444–55.

Ingram, R. (1991) Why does nursing need theory? *Journal of Advanced Nursing*, **16**, 350–3.

Jennings, B.M. (1987) Nursing theory development: success and challenges. *Journal of Advanced Nursing*, **12**, 63–9.

Jolley, M. and Allan, P. (eds) (1989) *Current Issues in Nursing*, Chapman & Hall, London.

Kolb, D.A. (1984) *Experimental Learning*, Prentice Hall, New Jersey.

Lancaster, J. (1985) The perils and joys of collaborative research: what to look for and what to avoid when putting together a research team. *Nursing Outlook*, **33**(5), 231–2, 238.

Leddy, S. and Pepper, J.M. (1985) *Conceptual Bases of Professional Nursing*, J.B. Lippincott, Philadelphia.

Marquis Bishop, S. (1986) Theory development process, in *Nursing Theorists and Their Work*, 2nd edn, (ed. A. Marriner), C.V. Mosby, St Louis.

Marriner, A. (ed.) (1986) *Nursing Theorists and Their Work*, 2nd edn, C.V. Mosby, St Louis.

McCafferey, M. (1979) *Nursing Management of the Patient with Pain*, 2nd edn, J.B. Lippincott, Philadelphia.

McCaugherty, D. (1991) The theory–practice gap in nurse education: its causes and possible solutions. Findings from an action research study. *Journal of Advanced Nursing*, **16**, 1055–61.

McCaugherty, D. (1992) The concepts of theory and practice. *Senior Nurse*, **12**(2), 29–33.

Meerabeau, L. (1992) Tactic nursing knowledge: an untapped resource or a methodological headache? *Journal of Advanced Nursing*, **17**, 108–12.

Melia, K. (1987) *Learning and Working: The Occupational Socialization of Nurses*, Tavistock, London.

Mintzberg, H. (1973) *The Nature of Managerial Work*, Harper and Row, London.

Newell, A. and Simon, H.A. (1972) *Human Problem Solving*, Prentice Hall, New Jersey.

Orem, D.E. (1985) *Concepts of Practice*, 3rd edn, McGraw Hill, New York.

Polanyi, M. (1958) *Personal Knowledge: Towards a Postcritical Philosophy*, Routledge and Kegan Paul, London.

Rafferty, A.M. and Hardy, L. (1982) Preaching and practising. *Nursing Times*, **78**(36), 1521–2.

Robinson, J.J.A. (1992) Problems with paradigms in a caring profession. *Journal of Advanced Nursing*, **17**, 632–8.

Roper, N., Logan, W. and Tierney, A. (eds) (1983) *Using a Model for Nursing*, Churchill Livingstone, London.

Russell, B. (1967) *The Problems of Philosophy*, Oxford University Press, Oxford.

Sbaih, L.C. (1992a) *Accident and Emergency Nursing: A Nursing Model*, Chapman & Hall, London.

Sbaih, L.C. (1992b) Finding a model that fits: the use of nursing models in A and E. *Professional Nurse*, 7(9), 566–9.

Sbaih, L.C. (1992c) *An Ethnographic Study of a Group of A and E Nurses*, unpublished dissertation, Manchester Metropolitan University.

Silva, M.C. (1986) Research testing nursing theory: state of the art. *Advances in Nursing Science*, 9(1), 1–11.

Sisk, H.L. and Williams, J.C. (1981) *Management and Organization*, 4th edn, South Western Publishing Company, Dallas.

Stevenson, O. (1974) Knowledge for social work. *British Journal of Social Work*, 1(2), 225–37.

United Kingdom Central Council (1992) *Code of Professional Conduct*, 3rd edn, UKCC, London.

Walsh, M. and Ford, P. (1989) *Nursing Rituals: Research and Rational Actions*, Heinemann Nursing, London.

Webb, C. (1986) Nursing models: a personal view. *Nursing Practice*, 1(4), 208–12.

Whitehead, G. (1978) *Business and Administrative Organization Made Simple*, W.H. Allen, London.

Whitis, G. (1985) Simulation in teaching clinical nursing. *Journal of Nursing Education*, 24(4), 161–3.

CHAPTER 8

The moral problems involved in the concept of patient triage in the A and E department

C. Jones and G. Hall

INTRODUCTION

Nursing triage in A and E continues to enjoy a high profile. It has been accepted within many departments and has become the subject for much debate, discussion and documentation within the nursing press. Despite its extensive coverage there has been very little exploration of underlying issues and instead emphasis has been placed on the organization, logistics and the apparent merits or demerits of implementing nursing triage in A and E.

Without berating such work, this chapter seeks to offer an alternative view of triage. The focus of the chapter is the examination of moral and ethical issues surrounding the current use of triage in A and E nursing. In addition there is also an attempt to explore assumptions about patients, many of which may be hidden but still influence decisions about prioritization in A and E.

The chapter offers access of information to all A and E nurses although parts of it may assume some background knowledge of philosophical principles. The reader is advised to take parts of the chapter and support reading with supplementary texts or group discussions where necessary.

The strength of this chapter lies in its encouragement of debate and potential challenge to the way in which traige systems are introduced and information should guide readers to make decisions about the future use of triage both in individual departments and in A and E on a national level. The use of case studies illustrates ideas and themes put forward and discussion points in the format of questions should help the reader to take the debate further.

The chapter may be used as a dip-in chapter or read from start to finish. It also offers a basis for the reading of other chapters in this book, for triage is a theme that has emerged within the book as a whole. In addition it sets the scene for further reading of philosophy and consideration of its place in A and E clinical practice. As with all other chapters the reference list offers a wealth of additional information that will be of use to the reader when taking areas of the debate into their own area of clinical practice.

DEFINITIONS

The concept of triage dates back to the 17th century where it was used as a quality control measure in the sorting and classification of food produce such as coffee and vegetables. While in the hospital setting the word 'triage' carries a different meaning, it could still be argued that one of the main intentions of its proponents is the improvement in service quality by the use of grading and classification tools.

Despite its relatively new introduction into Accident and Emergency departments in the United Kingdom (Jones, 1988), triage has become more prominent in recent years. This is particularly so since 1990 which saw the setting up of the Royal College of Nursing Accident and Emergency Nursing Association which included 'the advancement of triage' in A and E departments as one of its main objectives (RCN, 1990).

The goals of triage within each department vary but the consensus appears to concentrate on several core elements. These include early patient assessment, priority rating, first aid control, initiation of diagnostic tests along with control of patient flow, control of infection and an opportunity to become more involved in health promotion. Inherent within this is the aim to improve overall communications and thereby enhance public relations (Bailey *et al.*, 1987). It is commonly recognized that 'triage helps to promote a safe environment' for the patient and as such is seen as an 'important aspect of management in the Accident and Emergency department' (Bailey *et al.*, 1987).

TRIAGE AND APPROPRIATENESS OF ATTENDANCE

One key area of patient management is long waiting times. According to Nuttall (1986), this is 'common throughout the world' and can be attributed, in part, to the problem of 'casual or inappropriate attendances' at A and E (Blythin, 1988). This begs the question of who exactly is an inappropriate attender. The decision to label individuals, along with the whole concept of prioritization of care, raises some fundamental questions of justice which are central to an examination of triage.

The issue of how to divide the resources allocated to health care and the problems produced by such decisions appear regularly in nursing and medical literature. This is particularly the case when discussing the dilemmas surrounding the allocation of dialysis machines or intensive care beds, but an area of health care where decisions involving the division of resources seem to have been accepted with the minimum of controversy or debate is that of A and E.

Points for discussion

- Is there any way around rationing health care resources? What if the government simply provided more cash? Would this solve the problem?

- Is the absence of controversy surrounding health resource allocation in A and E due to the fact that the decision making process, through triage system, is made explicit?

George (1976) considers that triage is a process in which the assessment of the patient determines the urgency of need in order to 'designate appropriate health care resources to care for the identified problem'. Nevertheless, it is certain that if there were unlimited resources in A and E a triage system would be superfluous and everyone would get whatever treatment they wanted when they wanted it. It is a contemporary truism that health resources are finite and the demand for them is infinite and therefore the issue of how to divide scarce health care resources among equally deserving clients is one that is fraught with moral doubts and dilemmas.

How this division of resources is made and the problems that such decisions throw up will be discussed in this chapter. It will hopefully become clear that the problems associated with triage in A and E are at heart as complex as those in other, more high technology areas but the speed of decision making in A and E leaves little time or opportunity for reflection or consideration of the complex moral issues inherent within decisions to give to one patient and to deny another.

DESERTS AND NEEDS

In A and E, the widely accepted and perfectly serviceable principle of 'first come, first served' has to some extent been replaced by another principle which, though it is said to be fairer, is less comprehensible to the public as they fail to understand what that principle is and how it applies to them. This principle appears to have something to do with the level of need, but how that need is measured and whether those measurements contain all the considerations necessary is open to question.

Case study

A man attends his local hospital accompanying his son who thinks he may have broken his arm playing football. The son, 16, is in pain and complaining to the father. During their stay in the waiting room, they see a sequence of people arrive later than them but going in before them. The boy cannot understand why he is deliberately kept waiting while others, apparently less seriously injured than himself, are sped through. His father cannot explain why this should be so, nor can he obtain a satisfactory response from the triage nurse who, while telling the man that more serious cases are being seen first, cannot tell him what those cases are. His frustration at his long wait and his son's pain are therefore protracted.

Points for discussion

- Does nurse accountability stretch far enough to imply a duty on the triage nurse in this case to tell the man precisely why he is being kept waiting? If not, in what sense is this nurse accountable at all?

- Or does the countervailing principle of patient confidentiality hold sway? Is it not important that the triage system achieves credibility in the patient's eyes by convincing all the participants that need is actually being met and the prioritization is not entirely arbitrary?

A study conducted in 1976 by O'Flanagan suggested that over a six month period 2000 new attenders were seen at one A and E department. O'Flanagan's findings indicated that of that 2000, two-thirds could have been more appropriately treated by the general practitioner. But how and by whom is the appropriateness of someone's illness or condition measured? Cliff and Wood (1986) and Davidson *et al.* (1983) stated that one reason inappropriate attenders come to A and E is related to their own perception of their ailments, which some of them feel require urgent or immediate attention. Although education of patients in this area is advocated, the whole issue of treatment on a basis of need is brought into question – the question of whose need?

Point for discussion

● Have you ever heard the word 'rubbish' applied to the sort of cases that have presented in A and E? What does this expression mean? Does it represent a rough and ready statement of the seriousness of the patient's condition or something more judgemental about the patient?

TRIAGE IN DISASTER AND IN THE MILITARY: EQUALITY AND UTILITY

Traditionally it is believed that during the Crimean War a form of triage was introduced with a starkly utilitarian aim; soldiers adequately fit to fight were required in large numbers. The seriously injured were left to die whilst the less seriously injured were patched up and sent back to fight at the front. This was not the last time that this approach was to be taken in war. Young (1986) refers to the issue of need in his comments relating to the Second World War. Here the dilemma hinged on the use of antibiotics, which were in short supply. The American authorities decided to reserve penicillin for the treatment of soldiers who had contracted venereal diseases (VD) during leave rather than soldiers wounded in combat. Here the emphasis was focused on the concept of the common good where it was argued that those soldiers with VD could be treated more rapidly than those wounded. By treating these diseases first there would be more men available to fight and the prospect of an increased herd survival would be enhanced. This highlighted the conflict of the rights of the individual versus the good of the community. It was resolved in favour of the common good.

A similar principle may be considered to hold good in respect of major civilian disasters. Let us imagine the evacuation of casualties from a gas explosion site. Would it, for example, be appropriate to distribute ambulance places randomly with each person receiving an equal chance of going to hospital? Such a situation would certainly have the advantage of ensuring that there was equal treatment for all. But how far would you take equality? If it became clear that not everyone would have a place on the ambulances then would it be just to take equality to its logical conclusion and say that if everyone cannot go then no one should? It would guarantee equality of treatment but such a suggestion would have some very uncomfortable implications.

Our response to major disasters would appear to be fundamentally utilitarian. It is aimed at doing the maximum good for the maximum number. We are making the most out of a difficult if not tragic situation. But how is this best achieved?

The procedure adopted at such a disaster is essentially to form a queue. An individual's position in the queue is determined not by the time of arrival, as with queues in the post office, but more by the grading given to them by professionals in charge of the situation and subsequent evacuation. An individual's place in the queue varies according to the severity of their injury but this place may also be influenced by the severity of the injuries suffered by those discovered after them and to some extent by those who were discovered before them who have died and made a place available.

In general, though, their fate will be determined by whether the individual is likely to survive with minimal or extensive medical intervention or whether they are not likely to survive at all. Edwards (1989) states that 'experience in major civilian disasters avoids waste of valuable time on victims with little or no chance of survival' and the instances he highlighted are victims who have suffered 100% burns or even hypoxic cardiac arrest. In the heat of catastrophe, the aim is the evacuation of the greatest number as quickly as possible. To this end Edwards (1989) contends that 'public officials and slightly injured persons are selected for treatment before those who have been severely hurt'. The rationale in this case is that people in these first categories can effectively restore communication, transportation and order to a devastated area, without which further numbers may perish. The ultimate aim will then be to maximize the effectiveness of the resources available by removing to safety as many people as possible. Again the elements of a naked utilitarianism can be seen here with all its strengths and weaknesses. The aim is measurable maximization of welfare, even at the cost of disregarding the rights of the system's losers.

While this might appear to be a commonsense course of action, it has some serious implications. If it was felt that someone's condition was so serious and their need was so great that ensuring an ambulance place for them would obstruct the removal of many less seriously ill victims, would it be fair and just to give them priority? Or would it be better to hold on to that person in the hope that they survived and could be moved out later in order to move a greater number of victims during the initial stages? Or to put it another way – to whom do we owe the greater respect: the individual whose suffering and risk are greatest or the many whose needs are less severe and are easily met?

Points for discussion

●   If maximizing the numbers through the system is justifiable in war and in disasters, why not apply this principle in day-to-day practice? Allowing those who needed maximum attention to die would permit the majority of A and E attenders, the relatively fit, to be treated quicker and in greater numbers. It would also save enormous amounts of cash. Yet it seems a course of action which is repugnant. Why is this so, when in war it becomes standard practice?

● Would treating the less ill first complicate or simplify your own practice? How would you feel having to implement a military style triage system? Would you feel you were maximizing benefit or that you were hopelessly compromised?

One implication of any system of prioritizing care and attempting to target resources in line with social goals is, in the words of Young (1986), 'an upfront rejection of the principle of the independent and equal value of each human life'. Instead, the overriding concern is that of ensuring the common good.

Few question the justice of utilitarian approaches in circumstances of major civilian disaster despite the fact that there are some very problematic assumptions which underpin such a strategy. This is made clear when you consider that triage practice in a normal A and E department operates from fundamentally different moral premises.

If the disaster plan emphasizes the division of resources on a strictly utilitarian basis, the normal hospital triage principle is almost the reverse. In the normal event persons who are very sick or severely injured will have their rights respected and obtain maximum care and treatment whilst those who are less sick will be asked to wait until the sicker person's claims have been dealt with. Priority will not be based on herd survival calculated on numbers but on initial and continued assessment of the individual's needs. Their position in the queue is determined by these needs: the more their need, the higher up the priority ladder they rise.

It is perhaps even conceivable that victims of a major civilian disaster are assessed using both types of triage approaches in the one event. At the scene, assessment takes place where utilitarian considerations predominate. The decisions made may be responsible for the movement of the victim to an area where the notion of respect for the individual then takes precedence. In other words a seriously ill victim might find himself at the end of a queue at the scene of the incident and yet at the front of the queue on arrival at hospital. Somewhere on the way his status will change and the moral assumptions in his case will make a subtle but decisive shift.

Case study

A woman is one of the victims of a major motorway road traffic accident. She has witnessed some debate concerning another more seriously ill victim who was not considered fit for immediate transfer. On arrival at hospital she sees the same woman treated as a priority case, bypassing other less injured people who were given easier and quicker access to the ambulances at the scene of the accident. She cannot understand the logic of this conundrum; one minute the woman is considered an unsuitable candidate for an ambulance place and the next she is considered a prime candidate for priority care.

Point for discussion

● How can this shift in emphasis be justified? Isn't changing one's opinion quickly like this commonly referred to as hypocrisy? Would consistency of approach bring any advantages?

TRIAGE DECISIONS AND NON-HEALTH CONSIDERATIONS

There are of course many other issues involved in the triage decision. For example, if triage is basically about prioritization of scarce resources then surely we should take into account wider issues than just the nature of the injury presented.

Let us examine age as a determinant of need. Current triage systems will often include directions within their guidelines to give priority to the very young or the very old because of their perceived greater risk from mortality and morbidity. But other non-pathological life states will likewise predispose the patient to greater mortality or morbidity.

The Black Report published in 1980 and cited in *Inequalities in Health* (1988) by Townsend and Davidson produced figures on mortality and morbidity rates to identify areas of inequality of health in British society. Evidence suggested that the level of seriousness and the number of episodes of illness were adversely affected by a person's wealth and social standing and that the poorer classes tended to be sicker and die younger than the more affluent. Since the Report, further research has been undertaken which suggests that these trends have not changed: indeed *The Health Divide*, published in 1986 and also cited in *Inequalities in Health*, only serves to confirm the Black Report's findings. Therefore, any A and E admission for a poorer person may be of heightened consequences in terms of their risk to health. In spite of such suggestions no formal account is taken of this in the conventional triage process. In more specific terms the A and E triage system is not seen as having a role in making good the health deficits of society at large and so has no redistributive agenda in dividing its resources. A poorer person attending their local A and E for treatment of symptoms identical to those of a millionaire will receive no extra formal considerations for being poor even though they have come from and in some cases will go back to conditions which may ultimately predispose to the shortening of their life.

Case study

A man is admitted from a local council estate where there is a lot of unemployment and social deprivation. He has suffered a painful fracture of a number of ribs. He is thin and pale and his garments are shabby and old. In the next cubicle is a man who has been admitted from a nearby public school who has sustained an injury while playing rugby. He is healthy looking but in pain. His garments are new and in good repair.

Points for discussion

- Is there a case for arguing that the poorer man is a worse health risk, due to poor housing conditions and a lower health baseline, and that he deserves more access to available health care resources?

- Or are we obliged to be evenhanded to the extent that we make triage decisions exclusively on the immediate injuries presented?

- Is this approach evenhanded or is it closing our eyes to wider issues of health, thereby favouring the richer, more healthy person?

When it comes to age and gender, the 'women and children first' ethic is still represented in A and E in that a mother accompanied by young children is given priority and gains access to the system more rapidly than a young woman alone. However, when distributing resources there is generally little account taken of the duties the patient owes to his or her dependants.

Case study

A 32-year-old married woman with an 18-month-old baby is injured when the car she is travelling in is involved in a road traffic accident. The driver of the car is her friend aged 31 who has recently got engaged. Both women have sustained head and neck injuries of similar severity. Both receive the same assessment and are allocated resources accordingly with no provision being made for the fact that one woman has a young child dependent upon her and the other has not. This is what some would consider to be equality, but is the single woman actually equal? If we take a utilitarian view we could argue that the child should be given consideration as well as the mother and her prioritization could be justified in terms of the extra welfare thus ensured.

However, it is not clear how far this approach should be taken. Should the number of dependants be universally taken into account in making triage decisions? It is easy to imagine that a woman with a baby in her arms would be given priority: the baby is clearly visible and possibly audible. But should a man with three young children at home be given extra priority over a single and similarly injured man? Or what about a man with a demented and entirely dependent elderly mother? Would it be a fairer system of resource distribution to give people in this category extra access to emergency service, even if such a system were practicable?

Points for discussion

- Is the reason why wealth and social status are not taken into account because this would overcomplicate a system whose virtue is largely simplicity and speed?

- Think of your own practice. Even if desirable, would such a system be practicable? How would you go about constructing a system which compensated for poverty?

It seems, then, that the civilian triage process sees everyone as equal when racing for scarce A and E resources. It sees everyone competing from the same starting line with everyone having an equal amount of handicap. Nowhere in the triage process is there formal recognition of social factors to our disease processes and therefore there is no social compensation made in terms of increased access to facilities. Nor is there any recognition of anybody else's interest in an individual's survival and each individual's interest is seen to be equivalent to everyone else's.

HEALTH, RESPONSIBILITY AND TRIAGE DECISION MAKING

If poverty and family responsibilities do not count towards gaining triage points, are there any features of patients' lives which should be penalized? Young (1986) contends that there is 'no moral justification to make judgements about people' as our services should be rendered impartially 'without reference to race, colour, national background, worthiness or unworthiness or attractiveness or unattractiveness' of the people who seek our help. However, should account be taken of the patient's own contribution to their accident or illness when prioritizing patient care?

Case study

A 45-year-old man falls 10ft from a ladder in work and sustains facial lacerations involving the cheek, lip and nose. Admission to the A and E follows a 999 call which also brings in a man of similar age who is a 'regular' and as usual he is under the influence of alcohol. Possibly due to the alcohol he too has sustained facial injuries. Where all things are equal who should be seen by the facial surgeon first? Should the drunken man's behaviour be taken into account in terms of the injury being to some extent self-inflicted or should he gain more priority if we consider his social status and the fact that alcohol dependency syndrome is a sickness?

Is there a case for saying that some people contribute to their own sickness and some people are merely innocent victims of accidents? Chronic drug abuse, involvement in dangerous sports, persistent violent lifestyle all involve an element of conscious risk taking. Should part of the risk so taken be that, if there is an injury sustained, then the victim will be given a less favourable priority than a victim of a pure accident?

If we then take lifestyle into account when triaging, where do we draw the line? If limited resources are available, some may argue against giving people who live a morbid lifestyle an equal consideration with those whose illness has come upon them like a bolt from the blue.

Consider the cases of two people who are having difficulty breathing as a result of a severe chest infection. Both are cyanosed and are in extreme discomfort. The first smokes 20 cigarettes per day and the second smokes none. If they both were to need emergency anaesthetic in circumstances where there was only one anaesthetic machine, who should receive it? Now imagine the same situation where one smokes 80 cigarettes per day and the other only smokes 20. Which one now deserves the care and attention first?

Such a question is a difficult one to answer and most would like to think that their assessment would be impartial. But how impartial could one be if the situation arose where the innocent victim of a joyrider received less priority than the joyrider who caused the injuries in the first place? Even if such an impartial decision is easily justified in the minds of the health care professionals who base their considerations on sound clinical judgement, such a judgement would be, at best, difficult to justify to the victim's family and friends on any grounds.

On the other hand, if lifestyle considerations were to come into the triage process it would be virtually impossible to know where to stop. Smokers and people suffering from alcohol dependency syndrome are primary groups which can be readily picked on but what about people who indulge in contact sports and who regularly require extensive orthopaedic resources? Giving their claim less priority because they contributed to their own illness may raise as many problems as it solves. Similarly two people with chest pain might have indistinguishable clinical history, but to give one more priority because he did take regular exercise and therefore helped in some way to prevent his illness might leave many with an understandable sense of injustice and unfairness.

Points for discussion

- Are there no circumstances where it would be appropriate to restrict a person's access to health care because they create their own problems? If people claim the right to treatment, is there a corresponding duty to stay well?

- In your day-to-day practice, how do you feel about people whose admission is due to their own folly: the 'trivial' suicide attempt, the drunken driver and so forth? Do you feel that giving them the same access as others is just? Or do you think that discriminating against them would be an act of greater injustice?

ACCURACY OF TRIAGE DECISIONS AND NURSE ACCOUNTABILITY

So far the discussion has concentrated on whether the triage process is fair or unfair, just or unjust but has not considered the accuracy of triage decision making systems and the accountability of the nurse in discriminating between patients.

There are a number of different triage systems in operation at present, each with varying numbers and qualities of triage category. Read *et al.* (1992) state that in general, studies agree that nurse triage is 'safe and effective': an important finding to highlight. After all, in a system where the wrong decision can have catastrophic results, accuracy must be assured. The person responsible for decision making and priority setting will take both the moral and the legal accountability for any error. Accountability for mistakes is particularly relevant in a system where according to Pledge and Rock (1991), there was 'great variety in departments' implementation of triage, especially in training and record keeping'.

Even within an accurate system of prioritization there will still be room for interpretation and discretion. Bergman (1982) recognized that:

> Evaluation in nursing is a combination of objective measurement of concrete phenomena, as well as subjective perceptions and opinions on the 'feelings' of care as reported by recipients, providers and important others. After all, we are all fallible and susceptible to making judgements which are based on prejudice.

As an example of this phenomenon we might consider the work of Clayton and Davies (1982) who point out that 'There is a real danger that in a desire to be objective the easily measured aspects come to dominate', whilst the more intangible, 'the more difficult to identify but crucially important issues are played down or ignored'.

Either way, this point poses moral problems for the triage officer for, if the triage system chosen is very objective and rigid, then the triage officer may not be justified in discriminating between the nuances of patient details. This may give the nurse an organizational screen behind which to hide, but it may equally make the nurse a participant in an inaccurate system of prioritization which does not do justice to the complexities of day-to-day reality.

On the other hand, if the system chosen is fluid and flexible and allows the triage nurse the scope to use discretion and judgement then it will also allow the possibility of making a grave error of judgement for which there will be no one else to share responsibility. Not only will the scope for error possibly be opened up, but the accountability for such an error will be more focused on the individual decision maker.

THE MORALITY OF NOT TRIAGING PATIENTS

So far the concentration has been on the moral problems associated with the introduction and continued use of a triage decision making system. The final and possibly most important discussion must refer to the moral cost of not utilizing a system of triage prioritization on emergency victims. In fact, it is unlikely that an Accident and Emergency unit exists where some system of patient discrimination does not take place. It is hard to imagine anywhere where a person attending with, say, a fractured metacarpal would be admitted ahead of a person with central chest pain simply because they arrived in the department first.

Triage decision making, official or unofficial, will always be a feature of Accident and Emergency work. The point about an official triage system, with policies clearly outlined and publicized, is that the issues at stake in patient prioritization are made upfront and do not radically alter when the staff change over. An unofficial, gut feeling type of triage will carry no checks and balances against subjective biases. It will be subject to non-rational influences which would be less organizationally accountable. The public could scarcely have confidence in a system which was subject to wide differences and inconsistencies in emergency decisions. More than that, an unofficial and wholly subjective prioritization system provides no yardstick against which triage decisions could be evaluated in terms of outcome.

The inability effectively to evaluate treatment decisions which would be the consequence of a non-rational system of decision making might have the following moral consequences:

1. It may result in a net increase in suffering in that, while some may be advantaged by triage mistakes, the burden of errors would be borne by the most seriously ill. Gut feeling gone wrong could therefore produce an increase in deaths and sickness and with it a utilitarian deficit.
2. It may likewise result in a less efficient use and distribution of resources, both material and human, and therefore a reduction in the overall amount of help available to people in need.

A non-rational informal approach to triage may likewise result in a reduction in the amount of respect given to patients' rights and in the respect which is their due. A spurious equality may be shown to people of unequal need or vice versa. Not only that, but patients so disadvantaged may expect little in the way of accountability. With no formal decision making priority system in place, the hapless patient would have no standard of good practice against which to base a complaint. The only solid object against which to press a claim would be the professional judgement of the triage officer – a notoriously difficult task to perform.

FINAL THOUGHTS

The introduction of triage into Accident and Emergency departments has been welcomed as a new and rational system of emergency care delivery. However, its implementation has not been greeted with the sort of controversy that resource allocation decisions have induced in other areas of health care provision.

This is not to say that there are no difficult moral decisions implicit in the establishment of a triage process. It would be a mistake to imagine that patient prioritization is a problem-free approach. There are difficulties associated with the accountability of triage practitioners, as well as with the inability of triage systems to take into account relevant health care details such as dependants and social class.

Similarly, problems associated with triage extend into the relative priority given to patients whose contributory negligence has caused their health problems against those whose emergency is entirely fortuitous and unpredictable.

These issues, among others, together constitute a complex system of moral dilemmas which have surprisingly received little attention in the literature of emergency care, while in the field of access to high tech facilities they are well-rehearsed subjects of debate. It is to be hoped that an increased interest in the ethics of patient prioritization may lead ultimately to greater clarity on some of these thorny problems.

REFERENCES

Bailey, A., Hallam, K. and Hurst, K. (1987) Triage on trial. *Nursing Times*, **83**(44), 65–6.

Bergman, R. (1982) Evaluation of nursing care – could it make a difference? *International Journal of Nursing Studies*, **19**(2), 53–60.

Blythin, P. (1988) Triage documentation. *Nursing*, **3**(32), 32–4.

Clayton, S. and Davis, J.M. (1982) Value judgements. *Health & Social Service Journal*, **June** 776–7.

Cliff, K.S. and Wood, C.A. (1986) A & E Services – the ambulant patient. *Hospital & Health Service Review*, **82**(2), 74–7.

Davidson, A.G., Hildrey, A.C. and Floyer, M.A. (1983) Use and misuse of an A & E department in East End of London. *Journal of Royal Society of Medicine*, **76** 37–40.

Edwards, J.D. (1989) Mass casualties. *British Journal of Hospital Medicine*, **42**, 99.

George, J.E. (1976) Emergency nurse beware. *Emergency Nurse Legal Bulletin*, **Winter**.

Jones, G. (1988) Top priority. *Nursing Standard*, **3**(7), 28.

Nuttall, M. (1986) The chaos controller. *Nursing Times*, **82**(20), 66–8.

O'Flannagan, P. (1976) The work of an A & E Dept. *Journal of the Royal College of General Practitioners*, **26**, 54–60.

Pledge, M. and Rock, D. (1991) Priorities of care for the walking wounded. *Professional Nurse*, **May**, 463–5.

Read, S., George, S. and Williams, B. (1992) Piloting an evaluation of triage. *International Journal of Nursing Studies*, **29**(3), 275–88.

Royal College of Nursing A & E Forum (1990) *A & E Nurse Practitioner Guidelines*, RCN, London.

Townsend, P. and Davidson, S. (1988) *Inequalities in Health: The Black Report and the Health Divide*, Penguin, Harmondsworth.

Young, W.D. (1986) Current ethical issues in emergency care. *Journal of Emergency Nursing*, **12**(5), 301–4.

CHAPTER 9

The elderly person in A and E

P. Kingston and A. Hopwood

INTRODUCTION

Using the term 'elderly' is fraught with stereotypes and myths which may affect how nurses perceive elderly persons. This is an important issue to debate for elderly people will increasingly form a large section of the population of A and E.

Before starting this chapter the reader is advised that there is unique information to be gleaned, all of which is suitable for consideration in the A and E department. The chapter aims to explore a number of issues associated with the care of the elderly. In particular it aims to consider the myths and stereotypes associated with elderly persons both in society and in the A and E department. In addition two other areas of growing concern relating to elderly people will be examined: alcohol abuse by the elderly and abuse and neglect of the elderly. A theme running through this chapter is that elderly people are not a homogeneous group and as a result they require suitable assessment and intervention. It is not enough to know about the care of the adult to satisfactorily care for the elderly client.

This chapter is like many in the book; it can offer only a taster of some of the issues surrounding elderly persons. Points for discussion, in the form of questions in the text, should help the reader to consider specific areas of the chapter. It is then considered the responsibility of the reader to follow up ideas and develop the debate in their own area of clinical practice. To do this, it is assumed that the reader will make use of other supplementary texts to help consider themes and issues put forward.

References at the end of the chapter provide a wealth of additional information of which readers may wish to take advantage. Please note that Appendix 2 and Appendix 3 at the end of the book illustrate points raised in this chapter.

The proportion of elderly people in Britain has increased from 5.1% of the population in 1911 to 15.9% in 1991. Predictions suggest that the elderly population of 65 years and above will be 15.2% in 2001. However, of this total population, which will slightly decrease, the 75 or over population will increase from 6.9% to 7.1% and the 85 or over group from 1.4% to 1.8% (OPCS, 1984). This population change will have a profound effect on health service demand and the subsequent interventions elders will receive from nurse practitioners in the Accident and Emergency department.

DEMOGRAPHIC CHANGES, HEALTH STATUS AND GENDER

The demographic data above already suggest how difficult it is to talk of an 'elderly population'. Firstly, this population may include people from 55 to 95 years. Indeed, some 65-year-old individuals may be looking forward to 30 or more years in retirement. This wide age range of elderly people has caused social gerontologists to reconsider the definition of age and terms like 'old old' are used to signify people of 85 years and above.

The second important factor to consider alongside the age of the individual is the previous health status. Differences in mortality and morbidity are intrinsically bound to socioeconomic status. Indeed a male infant in social class I has a life expectation of 72.19 years compared to 65.02 years for his counterpart in social class V (Hart, 1990). Alongside life expectancy, morbidity differences are also found between men in social classes I and V. Townsend (1988) notes that in 65 of the 78 disease categories for men the standard mortality ratio for social classes IV and V were higher than either social class I or II. Victor (1980) suggests that these health differentials continue into the oldest age groups. Furthermore an Age Concern survey (1974) found that only 9% of elderly people in social classes I and II were severely restricted and dependent compared with 22% among unskilled and semiskilled groups.

Thirdly, there are gender differences in longevity, with women living longer than men. The gender ratio for people aged 65–69 is 121 (100 men for every 121 women) at 85 years and above this rises to 100 men/325 women. This does not suggest that women are healthier than men; in fact, Victor (1987) reports 'At all ages females demonstrate a higher level of disability than males'. This point is particularly important when discharge is being considered.

Point for discussion

● Discuss how different levels of disability may affect elderly people.

The demographic and health status research considered thus far suggests a highly variable picture of health amongst elderly people. It is therefore important that nurses do not perceive age necessarily as a period of health decline. Even though physical and mental frailty increase with age (Martin *et al.*, 1988), nurses must be aware that chronological age is not a valid predictor of health status. Nurses may see relatively healthy individuals at all ages from 55 to 95. Alternatively, relatively unhealthy individuals may be seen at 55 years and above. What is also important is the individual's capacity to adapt to changing health status. The knowledge and skill to evaluate the elderly person's ability to cope with the health or social problem that caused admission to the Accident and Emergency department is also crucial.

STEREOTYPES AND AGEISM

One of the major criticisms levelled at the nursing profession by social gerontologists concerns its orientation towards the social pathology of ageing. Wells (1980) notes that nurses she studied were 'a product of a training system that taught them a series of tasks and neglected to provide adequate information about care of the elderly'.

It is also possible that because nurses consistently care for elderly individuals who have health deficiencies, they begin to perceive all elderly people as having health deficiencies. It is clearly unacceptable to automatically assume that any elderly individual has sensory or health deficiencies solely because of the ageing process. All elderly people should be considered to have full sensory and health capacity until an assessment suggests otherwise. Nurses can sometimes be seen taking the history of an injury from a relative whilst talking about, and not to, the elderly patient – the 'does he take sugar?' phenomenon. The concept of stereotyping allied to ageism must also be considered alongside triage.

Points for discussion

- How do stereotypes of elderly people affect nursing interventions?
- Do nurses triage by age and not presenting condition?

Fries and Crapo (1981) suggest that:

When people develop cardiovascular or malignant disease in their 80s and 90s instead of their 50s and 60s, therapeutic and diagnostic decisions should be more humane and less dramatic.

Bytheway and Johnson (1990) comment that this may be considered 'a euphemistic way of proposing a policy of passive euthanasia, not for those who choose it, but rather for those over a certain age'.

Clearly nurses must proactively challenge those negative value judgements about elderly people that are apparent within health care settings. Triage must therefore be based solely on an evaluation of presenting trauma and injury, leaving value judgements about individuals aside.

REASONS FOR ATTENDANCE AT THE ACCIDENT AND EMERGENCY DEPARTMENT

The Accident and Emergency department is a place that seldom closes. It is often therefore the entry point for elderly people with social problems as well as for those requiring medical intervention. McDonald and Abrahams (1990) suggest that the elderly as a group attend Accident and Emergency departments because they know where it is and appreciate that they will be treated as soon as they arrive for care. Many elderly patients value their independence and will try to manage at home with little outside help. Evidence suggests that over 90% of the elderly live at home and want to remain there (McDonald and Abrahams, 1990). It can therefore be appreciated that when elderly patients present to the Accident and Emergency department they are often very ill with a multitude of problems – physical, psychological and social. Visiting the Accident and Emergency department is extremely worrying for the elderly patient and this anxiety (Clark, 1991; Sbaih, 1992) may exacerbate the presenting condition.

Assessing sensory status

The Accident and Emergency department may be a frightening and unfamiliar place to many patients and this is especially so for the elderly. Clearly any degree of sensory impairment, visual or auditory, combined with anxiety will make the Accident and Emergency department a very daunting environment. In addition to the unfamiliar environment and fear of the unknown, the elderly patient may consider that because of their condition they will never leave hospital and will subsequently lose their independence. Reassurance will clearly be necessary that their condition will be dealt with promptly and a speedy rehabilitation will follow.

Skilled assessment of the elderly patient in the Accident and Emergency department should include an evaluation of the physical problems alongside the psychological and social problems. Certainly much relevant information will be supplied by the ambulance personnel. The nurse should also ascertain:

- what were the patient's home conditions?
- was it heated?
- what type of accommodation was it – single storey/double/warden controlled?

The responses to all these questions will assist the nurse to construct a mental picture of the elderly person's home circumstances. This knowledge is of vital importance when a discharge plan is being formulated in preparation for the patient's departure home from the Accident and Emergency department. The Accident and Emergency nurse can also acquire much information about the patient's health status and lifestyle when a full body examination has been completed. The nurse also needs to discover the status of the patient's activities of daily living (ADL), including shopping, meals, hygiene, and if they require support, who provides it?

This information may help to frame the diagnosis but may also influence postdischarge interventions. When the condition of the patient requires that they be undressed the general condition of the skin can be evaluated and noted. Communication with the patient throughout all interventions will also gather information about the lifestyle and degree of intervention likely after discharge, if any is required. Accident and Emergency departments are busy environments, with a bustling atmosphere (Walsh, 1990). It is apparent that if patients sense this busy atmosphere around them, they may feel themselves to be a 'nuisance' and will therefore not talk as freely and as openly as they would if they felt that the nurse dealing with them was not quite so rushed (Bradley and Edinberg, 1990). It is extremely important that the nurse in the Accident and Emergency department is aware of the need to spend time with the elderly patient in order to obtain relevant information.

Nurses must make a conscious effort to spend time with the elderly patient in the light of research suggesting that in fact nurses spend very small amounts of time talking to the elderly (Wells, 1980). Bradley and Edinberg (1990) also suggest that technical language and jargon used when questioning patients can confuse them and so lead to inappropriate responses. When talking to elderly patients it is therefore vital that the nurse communicates without using jargon or technical terms so that the patient understands the questions and what is required of them. This encourages feedback from the patient and ensures that all information that has been given has been understood. Talking to the elderly patient will also give the Accident and Emergency nurse some objective information about sensory status; for example, can the patient hear what is being said to them? Degenerative changes within the ear do increase in the elderly (Whitbourne, 1985) and therefore hearing is often of poorer quality than that of the younger patient. Despite this, it is imperative that the nurse does not automatically assume that the elderly person's hearing is impaired. Slow, clear speech in full view of the patient to enable lip reading to take place (Walsh, 1990) and a check to ensure that any hearing aid is in full working order will clearly be necessary and enhance communication with the elderly patient. Clark (1991) suggests that elderly people:

> ... often complain that they are unable to understand rather than not being able to hear ... this difficulty ... is usually experienced initially when the environment is noisy or when speech is rapid.

With this caveat in mind the nurse must not confuse the ability to comprehend what is said with a hearing impairment. In addition to the degenerative changes which take place in the ear, elderly patients may also experience a deterioration in their sight. This must be accounted for in the nurse's assessment of the elderly patient. For example, do they wear spectacles and if so, have they brought them to the department with them? If the nurse suspects a degree of visual impairment an introduction may be necessary as the patient may be unaware of her presence. The nurse must then find the best position in which to communicate, usually directly in front of the person at the same facial height (Koshy, 1989). The nurse must also assess the elderly patient's psychological state in order to be aware of their normal functioning level. The nurse needs to be cognisant of the normal mental state of the patient before admission, especially if the patient shows signs of confusion.

Points for discussion

- What special techniques may be required in order to communicate with older people?

- How can jargon and technical terms be avoided during the communication process?

Questioning of any individuals, especially relatives or carers accompanying the patient, may provide the nurse with an account of the psychological status of the elderly person. The importance of knowing the elderly patient's previous mental state cannot be overemphasized because confusion can often be a symptom of hypoxia due to a chest infection or unstable diabetes mellitus. Other factors that must be considered include drug toxicity, including digitalis, hypnotics and Parkinson's disease medication, and disorientation because of the environment. The stress and anxiety of being brought to the Accident and Emergency department and then perhaps being placed in a cubicle without any visual stimulation may confuse the elderly person (Walsh,

1990). It is therefore important that the nurse consistently informs the elderly person of where they are and what is going to happen to them.

Point for discussion

● How can information be used to alleviate anxiety during and after admission to the Accident and Emergency department?

Falls

It has been suggested that approximately one-third of elderly people experience one or more falls during a 12 month period (Bowling and Grant, 1992). Statistics also suggest more than 300 000 people aged 65 and over attend Accident and Emergency departments each year in England and Wales as a result of accidents and the majority of these attendances are caused by falls (Bowling and Grant, 1992).

Causes of falls in the elderly include accidental falls, for example slipping, falling over objects and loose carpets, and also falls caused by physiological changes including transient ischaemic attacks, vertigo, central nervous system degeneration, postural hypotension and weakness in the legs (Morfitt, 1983). The incidence of patients sustaining a fractured neck of femur has increased to such an extent that it almost justifies the term 'epidemic' (Royal College of Physicians, 1989). Many Accident and Emergency departments see an elderly person after they have sustained a fall resulting in a fractured neck of femur on average once a day (Walsh, 1990). Versluysen (1986) studied the management of patients with a fractured neck of femur and found that 66% developed pressure sores, demonstrating that long periods of time spent on hard trolleys in the Accident and Emergency department predisposed these patients to the development of pressure sores. It is therefore extremely important that patients with a high risk of pressure sores receive frequent nursing care.

Point for discussion

● How can time spent waiting on trolleys in the Accident and Emergency department be reduced?

Pain

Pain threshold is unchanged by age. However, Cummings (1991) suggests that many elderly patients are hesitant to report pain. The Accident and Emergency nurse should therefore observe the patient's facial expressions and vital signs for evidence of pain, although it is important to note that certain behavioural cues, moaning and wincing may not be present in milder pain (Stewart, 1977). Analgesia according to the patient's individual requirements should be administered and its effectiveness documented, with special consideration of the sensitivity of the elderly to opiates.

The maxim to follow with all patients should be based on Mc-Caffery's (1972) definition: 'Pain is whatever the experiencing person says it is, existing whenever he says it does'.

Point for discussion

● Is pain management influenced by stereotypes about older people?

Hypothermia

Sadly elderly people are sometimes brought to Accident and Emergency departments suffering from hypothermia. This is a particularly disturbing fact in a wealthy Western society and comparisons with other countries suggest the United Kingdom fares very badly. Levels of cold related deaths total 11% in Scotland, 4–6% in France, Sweden, USA and Canada, with overall UK rates measuring 12% (Grut, 1987).

Points for discussion

● What are the circumstances which lead to hypothermia?

● Has the patient any other illnesses which may predispose the individual to the hypothermia?

The ageing process

There is no doubt that physiological changes occur with age (Whitbourne, 1985) but the variability between individuals must always be considered. Every system in the body is affected by ageing in some way and a brief understanding of these changes can help the Accident and Emergency nurse to be more sensitive to the potential problems and limitations affecting the elderly. It is also important that the nurse allows the elderly person dignity and empowerment; if the older person can get undressed the nurse should not intervene even if undressing may take the elderly person several minutes. The nurse must make a conscious effort to spend time with the elderly person, allowing them to proceed at their own pace. A professional maxim to follow is suggested by McDonald and Abrahams (1990):

> The attitude of emergency department staff toward the elderly should reflect respect for the autonomy of the individual and an awareness of the patient's role in the decision making.

Point for discussion

● How can an elderly person's dignity and autonomy be enhanced in the Accident and Emergency department?

It has already been suggested that the nurse should speak clearly and relatively slowly when talking to a patient. Checks on the hearing aid, if used, should be made and the patient questioned about their understanding of the contents of the conversation. Confusion is sometimes identified as a problem when dealing with elderly people. The confusion may be due to a progressive condition like dementia or a psychological state which is brought about by changes in physical or environmental factors, such as sudden and unexpected hospitalization, especially when this is caused by various disease processes. Hypoxia, hypothermia, electrolyte imbalance and uncontrolled diabetes mellitus may cause significant confusion in an elderly patient (Walsh, 1990). The causes of confusion, whether acute or chronic, would appear to be self-explanatory, if not always easy to diagnose.

Alcohol abuse

Attention is now being drawn to the significant health problem of alcohol abuse which affects elderly people and can cause confusion, falls and malnutrition (Malcolm, 1992). It has been documented that alcohol abuse by elderly people may be overlooked because the impairment caused by alcohol may be attributed to the ageing process (Iliffe, 1991). Degenerative changes in the nervous system, especially in those areas which control balance, will enhance the patient's sensitivity to alcohol. Consequently a wide range of problems caused by excessive alcohol ingestion can be exacerbated in the elderly (Black, 1990).

Problem drinking is most certainly not often recognized and can be very carefully hidden in the elderly in comparison with their younger counterparts. This may be due to the fact that it can be attributed to inadequate adjustment to changes in later life, such as retirement, bereavement, ill health or loneliness. Alcohol abuse is traditionally seen as a problem of middle-aged men (Hartford and Samorajski, 1982) and identifying alcohol abuse as a problem and separating the social consequences of abuse from those related to ageing is difficult. Little has been written on the topic of alcohol consumption by elderly people (Dunne and Shipperheijn, 1989). Therefore the aim of the inclusion of this topic is to promote thought and discussion about the subject of alcohol abuse in the elderly. The application of this knowledge concerning the growing problem of alcohol abuse may assist the nurse to deliver appropriate physical and psychological care to the elderly patient. It has been stated that one elderly person in ten has a drink problem (Malcolm, 1992) and that at least 10% of patients presenting with dementia have alcohol related brain disease (Dunne and Shipperheijn, 1989). These facts suggest that nurses working in the Accident and Emergency department must have at some point encountered an elderly person with an alcohol problem.

Point for discussion

● Are nurses aware of the growing problem of alcohol abuse amongst elderly people?

Elderly alcohol misusers are more likely than younger misusers to hide their drinking and they have a tendency to drink daily rather than to binge (Dunne and Shipperheijn, 1989). This may explain why, if an elderly alcohol abuser is brought into the Accident and Emergency department, they may be diagnosed as 'confused', especially if they have built up a tolerance to alcohol. When dealing with or trying to identify an elderly alcohol abuser it is important to understand the effects that alcohol has on elderly people and the problems abuse can cause. Medical problems tend to be more prominent in elderly alcohol abusers compared with their younger counterparts. This is due to the reduction in total body water and lean body mass which occurs with ageing. This accounts for a higher blood alcohol concentration in the elderly than in younger people. The rate of blood flow through an ageing liver also decreases, therefore rapid metabolism of alcohol in the body is reduced. Musculoskeletal pain, insomnia, loss of libido, depression and anxiety are recognized complications of heavy drinking, but are also common complaints among the elderly population. It is therefore necessary to differentiate symptoms caused by alcohol abuse from symptoms caused by the ageing process. Small amounts of alcohol (less than two units) can cause central nervous system problems (Black, 1990) which can lead to an increased incidence of confusion and falls. Other medical problems caused by alcohol abuse include accidental hypothermia, hypoglycaemia, incontinence, malnutrition, peripheral neuropathies and liver disease.

Point for discussion

● Is alcohol abuse considered as a cause for falls and confusion in older people?

It is suggested that many men and women drink silently at home and go out only for more supplies (Jacobson, 1983). This may explain why relatives and friends are not necessarily aware of excessive alcohol consumption. Interactions between alcohol and prescribed drugs may also induce problems. 'Compliance with multiple drug regimes, often encountered in the elderly, is found to be difficult enough when sober' (Malcolm, 1992).

Mental health problems are also commonly related to alcohol abuse, particularly in elderly people (Malcolm, 1992) and the safe operation of household appliances such as kettles and electric blankets can be dangerous under the influence of alcohol. Malcolm suggests that death from house fires is related to alcohol abuse in elderly people. There does appear to be a vicious circle of isolation, depression, ill health and bereavement and drinking is often the cause of this cycle. Alcohol is also an important factor in up to 30% of elderly suicides (Goddard and Gask, 1991). It is also important to note the addictive nature of alcohol and the social problems this addiction may intensify. Malcolm (1992) suggests that financial and social problems result from alcohol abuse. Elderly people do not usually have unlimited funds and therefore may spend money on alcohol instead of food and heating. Clearly elderly people have health deficiencies that can be exacerbated by alcohol abuse. They may present to the Accident and Emergency department with any one or a combination of these problems. The role of the nurse then includes a differentiation between what may be a health deficiency, alcohol abuse or indeed a combination of both.

Elder abuse and neglect

Within the last ten years the discovery of elder abuse and neglect in the domestic setting has taken place. However, it is not considered a legitimated social problem of the magnitude of child abuse or spouse abuse in Britain. This is clearly not the case in America where elder abuse and neglect is considered a social problem in its own right, demanding legislation and intervention. In Britain we are slowly discovering that elderly people are abused and neglected in the domestic setting in which they are often being cared for. Nurses in Accident and Emergency departments do not usually consider injuries sustained by elderly people as non-accidental.

Points for discussion

- Do nurses consider whether an injury to an elderly person may have been non-accidental?

- Does the injury match the history from the patient?

- Does the injury match the history from the relative/carer?

These questions are always at the front of a mental checklist when children with injuries are admitted. It is important that nurses begin to ask the same questions about injuries to elders. Clearly one way of facilitating this type of analysis is to use policies and procedures (see Appendix 2).

Point for discussion

● Has the Accident and Emergency department a policy/ procedure to follow in suspected or known cases of elder abuse/neglect?

Policies and procedures enable a consistent evaluation of potential abusive and neglectful behaviours. The latest contribution from the Social Services Inspectorate (1993) *No Longer Afraid: The Safeguard of Older People in Domestic Settings,* suggests:

> The following staff may at some time be in a position to identify abuse ... community nursing staff and other health care staff, including those working in Accident and Emergency departments.

They can also provide education for those staff members who are not aware of the phenomenon of elder abuse and neglect. It is important to understand that at this point in time definitions do not necessarily help with the diagnosis of elder abuse and neglect. However, the eight categories found in definitions go some way to suggest what types of abuse and neglect occur. These include:

1. assault;
2. deprivation of nutrition;
3. administration of inappropriate drugs or deprivation of prescribed drugs;
4. emotional abuse;
5. sexual abuse;
6. deprivation of help in performing activities of daily living;
7. involuntary isolation and confinement;
8. financial abuse.

(Bennett and Kingston, 1993)

Research has suggested certain factors that can be associated with increased risk of abuse and these include:

1. Psychosocial history. Is there a history of alcohol abuse, drug abuse or mental illness among any of the carers?
2. Transgenerational violence. Is there a past history of violence in the family?
3. Dependency. Are any of the carers dependent upon the elderly person for income or shelter?
4. Stress. Have stressful life events occurred recently?

5. Isolation. Does the elderly person have a satisfactory amount of family contact?
6. Living arrangements. Does the elderly person share accommodation with their carer?

(Wolf and Pillemer, 1986)

When the potential forms of abuse are considered alongside the potential risk factors, a picture of 'at risk' situations begins to emerge. However, it is very difficult to discover elder abuse and neglect because elderly people are reluctant to report to professionals and professionals do not recognize the signs of elder abuse (Kosberg, 1988). Because practitioners are only just beginning to understand this latest discovery in the family violence domain, education is clearly important. Only when the social phenomenon of elder abuse receives as much time in the nursing/medical and social work curricula as child abuse will professionals begin to seriously consider how we can address the problem.

DISCHARGE CONSIDERATIONS

Discharge considerations are a crucial part of the Accident and Emergency nurse's role and will become even more important with the rapidly changing world of the National Health Service. Both *Caring for People* (Department of Health, 1989a) and *Working for Patients* (Department of Health, 1989b) will influence the mode of service provision. With the advent of trust status and fundholding general practitioners, entirely new relationships are being designed. It will be vitally important that the nurse who discharges the elderly patient is entirely confident that aftercare arrangements are satisfactorily prepared.

Rosenfield (1990) conducted a study of a group of elderly patients discharged after attending the Accident and Emergency department of a large Australian hospital. This study revealed that before-and-after comparisons of aspects of physical functioning revealed a considerable loss of independence in the period following the visit to the hospital. Subsequent hospital admission or death was observed in 30 of the 90 patients studied. This clearly suggests that elderly patients discharged from the Accident and Emergency department are at risk and require special consideration prior to discharge. This research suggested that documentation of social and physical problems and the actions taken should be improved. A study in Edinburgh (Currie et al., 1984) of 100 discharged elderly patients reported an increase in dependency in 52 of the cases, with 22 reporting a loss of outdoor activities, for example shopping, and a further 28 reporting loss of indoor activities including cooking and housework. When the records of these 100 patients were examined only 13 had any functions recorded other than range of joint movement. Support arrangements were recorded in only 17 cases, mental status in five cases and referral to the social worker in only nine cases.

It is therefore important to note Lukacs' (1991) suggestion that a 'geriatric nursing assessment form' is used to enhance the quality of care by providing a comprehensive assessment and establishing continuity of care. The authors agree with the suggestion, but advise a change of terms from 'geriatric' to 'elderly care'. An elderly care nursing assessment form would provide uniformity in assessing the needs and problems of the elderly patient attending the Accident and Emergency department. It has been recognized that the differing levels of knowledge and experience of individual nurses determine whether patient assessment is thorough or incomplete (Mathieson, 1988). The use of an assessment form would ensure that all aspects of the elderly patient's injury, problem, lifestyle and needs are assessed and such problems as possible alcohol abuse and elder abuse and neglect may be identified and acted upon. The form used should include personal and nursing information, it should provide easy reference to precise information, be simple to complete and therefore keep nursing time spent on documentation to a minimum (Mathieson, 1988). McInnes (1988) cautions that a significant reason for unsuccessful discharge of elderly people is because their initial problem was inadequately assessed and that incomplete rehabilitation was initiated following discharge. Harding and Modell (1989) state that the discharge from hospital of elderly patients is often 'poorly planned' and Victor and Vetter (1988) claim that discharge planning for the elderly is 'A very neglected aspect of patient care'.

The use of an elderly care nursing assessment form should enable a thorough and uniform assessment of the patient's needs and problems to take place and subsequent planning for discharge should follow using the data collected. Although preparation and planning for discharge is an integral aspect of the care of the elderly (Victor and Vetter, 1988), research suggests that preplanning does not always take place. Harding and Modell (1989), in a study of elderly people's experiences of discharge from hospital, found that 58% reported that their ability to cope at home had not been assessed prior to discharge. By assessing thoroughly the needs and problems of the elderly in the Accident and Emergency department, problems such as alcohol abuse, elder abuse and neglect, loneliness and depression may be identified and measures taken to help the elderly to cope. Harding and Modell (1989) suggest that on discharge home a letter should be sent to the patient's general practitioner. This should improve communication between the community and hospitals so that the optimum use of resources is made to support the elderly on their discharge. This is especially important now that the Community Care Act (DoH, 1989a) is in place.

It has been claimed that 'repeated visits to emergency departments are frequently caused by unresolved social problems which originated at the initial visit' (McDonald and Abrahams, 1990). A thorough pre-discharge report and elderly care nursing assessment form (see Appendix 2) may help to reduce repeated returns to the Accident and Emergency department. It may also be beneficial to include a copy of the elderly care nursing assessment form in order to highlight to the general practitioner any problems identified on the patient's visit to the Accident and Emergency department, for example, alcohol abuse, elder abuse and neglect and depression. This may assist general practitioners in the management of their elderly patients. This may certainly be the case with alcohol abuse, with Illiffe (1991) stating that 'General practitioners identify correctly only a minority of high-risk drinkers amongst their patients'.

A thorough and uniform assessment of the elderly and their problems in Accident and Emergency departments should subsequently lead on to a planned and successful discharge with relevant referrals made to the appropriate members of the primary care team. 'Accident and emergency departments have the obligation to provide a safe environment until a more appropriate setting is located' (McDonald and Abrahams, 1990).

Points for discussion

● How can discharge planning for elderly people be improved?

● What special arrangements may be necessary when considering discharge from the Accident and Emergency department for elderly people?

CONCLUSION

Demographic changes amongst the ageing population will clearly increase the numbers of elderly patients seen by nurses in the Accident and Emergency department. Accident and Emergency nurses will therefore need to be aware of the unique skills required to provide rapid, comprehensive, therapeutic interventions with elderly people. Knowledge of the myths and stereotypes that surround later life will help nurses to provide a person centred, individual assessment, avoiding value judgements based on ageism. A thorough understanding of the ageing process will help the nurse provide effective communication and an assessment that takes into account the 'normal ageing' process. Changes in the management of health services will require constant monitoring, followed by rapid adaptation of policies by the nurse in the Accident and Emergency department, especially when postadmission follow-up is being planned. Finally the recently discovered health and social problems of alcohol abuse and elder abuse and neglect will require careful consideration by Accident and Emergency nursing staff. New policies and guidelines will need to be devised to diagnose, monitor and intervene in cases of elder abuse and neglect.

REFERENCES

Age Concern (1974) *The Attitudes of the Retired and Elderly*, Age Concern, London.

Bennett, G. and Kingston, P.A. (1993) *Elder Abuse*, Chapman & Hall, London.

Black, D.A. (1990) Changing patterns and consequences of alcohol abuse in old age. *Geriatric Medicine*, **20**(1), 19–20.

Bowling, A. and Grant, K. (1992) Accidents in elderly care: a randomised controlled trial (part one). *Nursing Standard*, **6**(29), 28–30.

Bradley, J.C. and Edinberg, M.A. (1990) *Communication in the Nursing Context*, Appleton and Lange, California.

Bytheway, B. and Johnson, J. (1990) On defining ageism. *Critical Social Policy*, **29**, 5–27.

Clark, J.M. (1991) Communicating with Elderly People, in *Nursing Elderly People*, (ed. S.J. Redfern), Churchill Livingstone, London.

Cummings, J. (1991) Managing the patient with a fractured femur. *Nursing Standard*, **5**(25), 11–13.

Currie, C.T., Lawson, P.M., Robertson, C.E. and Jones A. (1984) Elderly patients discharged from an accident and emergency department – their dependency and support. *Archives of Emergency Medicine*, **1**, 205–13.

Department of Health (1989a) *Caring for People: Community Care in the Next Decade and Beyond*, CM 849, HMSO, London.

Department of Health (1989b) *Working for Patients*, CM 555, HMSO, London.

Dunne, F.J. and Schipperheijn, J.A.M. (1989) Alcohol and the elderly: need for greater awareness. *British Medical Journal*, **298**, 1660–1.

Fries, J.F. and Crapo, L.M. (1981) *Vitality and Ageing: Implications of the Rectangular Curve*, W.H. Freeman, San Francisco.

Goddard, C. and Gask, L. (1991) Problem drinking in the elderly: recognition and treatment. *Geriatric Medicine*, **21**(5), 18.

Grut, M. (1987) Cold-related deaths in some developed countries (letter). *Lancet*, **8525**, 212.

Harding, J. and Modell, M. (1989) Elderly people's experiences of discharge from hospital. *Journal of the Royal College of General Practitioners*, **39**(318), 17–20.

Hart, N. (1990) 'The sociology of health and medicine', in *Sociology: New Directions*, (ed. M. Haralambos), Causeway Press, England.

Hartford, J.T. and Samorajski, T. (1982) Alcoholism in the geriatric population. *Journal of the American Geriatrics Society*, **30**(1), 18–24.

Iliffe, S. (1991) Alcohol consumption by elderly people: a general practice study. *Age and Ageing*, **20**(2), 120–3.

Jacobson, S. (1983) Coping without alcohol. *Nursing Mirror*, **156**(6), 53–5.

Kosberg, J.I. (1988) Preventing elder abuse: identification of high risk factors prior to placement decisions. *The Gerontologist*, **28**(1), 43–50.

Koshy, K.T. (1989) I only have ears for you. *Nursing Times*, **85**(30), 26–9.

Lukacs, K.S. (1991) A geriatric nursing assessment form for the emergency department. *Journal of Emergency Nursing*, **17**(2), 86–9.

Malcolm, T. (1992) The demon drink. *Nursing the Elderly*, **4**(4), 22–4.

Martin J., Meltzer, H. and Elliot, D. (1988) *The Prevalence of Disability among Adults*, OPCS Surveys of Disability in Great Britain, Report No. 1, HMSO, London.

Mathieson, A. (1988) Rating needs. *Nursing Times*, **84**(35), 38–41.

McCaffery, M. (1972) *Nursing Management of the Patient with Pain*, J.B. Lippincott, Philadelphia.

McDonald, A.J. and Abrahams, S.T. (1990) Social emergencies in the elderly. *Emergency Medicine Clinics of North America*, **8**(2), 443–59.

McInnes, E.G. (1988) Failed discharges: setting standards for improvement. *Geriatric Medicine*, **18**(4), 35–42.

Morfitt, J.M. (1983) Falls in old people at home: intrinsic versus environmental factors in causation. *Public Health*, **97**, 115–20.

Office of Population, Censuses and Surveys (1984) *Census Guide No. 1*, HMSO, London.

Rosenfield, T. (1990) The fate of elderly patients discharged from the accident and emergency department of a general teaching hospital. *Community Health Studies*, **14**(4).

Royal College of Physicians (1989) Fractured neck of femur: prevention and management. *Journal of the Royal College of Physicians of London*, **23**(1), 8–12.

Sbaih, L. (1992) *Accident and Emergency Nursing*, Chapman & Hall, London.

Social Services Inspectorate (1993) *No Longer Afraid: The Safeguard of Older People in Domestic Settings*, HMSO, London.

Stewart, M.L. (1977) Measurement of clinical pain, in *Pain: A Source Book for Nurses and Other Health Professionals*, (ed. A.K. Jacox), Little Brown, Boston.

Townsend, P. (1988) *Inequalities in Health: The Health Divide*, Penguin, Harmondsworth.

Versluysen, M. (1986) How elderly patients with femoral fractures develop pressure sores in hospital. *British Medical Journal*, **292**, 1311–13.

Victor, C. (1980) *A Longitudinal Study of the Mortality of a 1% Sample of the Elderly in England and Wales*. Proceedings of the Annual Conference of the British Society for Gerontology, University of Aberdeen.

Victor, C. (1987) *Old Age in Modern Society: A Textbook of Social Gerontology*, Croom Helm, London.

Victor, C.R. and Vetter, N.J. (1988) Preparing the elderly for discharge from hospital: a neglected aspect of patient care. *Age and Ageing*, **17**(3), 155–63.

Walsh, M. (1990) *Accident and Emergency Nursing: A New Approach*, 2nd edn, Heinemann Nursing, Oxford.

Wells, T. (1980) *Problems in Geriatric Nursing Care,* Churchill Livingstone, Edinburgh.

Whitbourne, S.K. (1985) *The Aging Body,* Springer-Verlag, New York.

Wolf, R.S. and Pillemer, K.A. (1986) *Elder Abuse: Conflict in the Family,* Auburn House, Dover.

CHAPTER 10

Care of the child in the A and E department

R. Burton

INTRODUCTION

There are few A and E departments that do not have children as their clients. In addition, children form a large percentage of visitors of patients in A and E for a number of reasons. However, all experienced A and E nurses are happy with the care of children and their carers. Or are they?

This chapter will help the reader take that particular question further by exploring many known issues from a number of perspectives, all of which are introduced via the use of text and pictures, pictures that have been drawn by children visiting one particular A and E department and which aim to illustrate areas of care delivery and the environment through the eyes of the child.

The approach used in the chapter is to reintroduce much known information. This should allow the reader to reconsider the care of the child in A and E in terms of knowledge base and skills required. It is also acknowledged that the subject of children is enormous and it is impossible to cover all issues about children in the chapter. The reader may feel that important issues have been omitted; if so they are advised to read the chapter with reference to other supplementary texts. In addition the reader may feel that there is little new featured in the chapter; however, what is introduced allows the reader plenty of scope for the examination of ideas and themes within their own area of clinical practice.

Readers can enter all debates within the chapter through the use of discussion points, which take the form of questions directed at the reader. Discussion points should help the reader focus on particular parts of the chapter and consider information presented within their own department.

Themes running through the chapter include the child as a unique individual, the role of the nurse in the care of sick and well children in A and E and the specific role of the RSCN. As with all chapters, the answers remain with the reader following the consideration of ideas and perspectives. References at the end of the chapter contain much additional information which it is expected the reader will wish to tap into as required.

THE CHILD: AN INTRODUCTION

In 1746, the Earl of Chesterfield penned these words: 'The knowledge of the world is only to be acquired in the world and not in a closet'. (Chesterfield, 1979). In the child's quest for knowledge of the world he has been born into, his insatiable curiosity will often lead him into situations where he may be at risk of injury and even death. Because of their immaturity and their lack of experience, children are vulnerable to accidents (RCN, 1990). This combination of insatiable curiosity and limitless energy compels them to explore, to probe and to investigate the wonderful world they inhabit (Burton, 1993a). Wordsworth (1960) captures this child-like philosophy of the world in these beautiful words from his poem *Intimations of Immortality*:

> . . . delight and liberty, the simple creed
> of childhood, whether busy or at rest . . .

Children cannot be kept in closets, therefore accidents will happen to many children.

The word 'accident' implies a random event yet the existence of a higher risk group shows this is not entirely true (Graydon, 1989). Some factors which contribute to childhood accidents include:

- social factors;
- the inherent nature of a child;
- the lack of adequate adult supervision;
- environmental risk and poverty;
- stress;
- the lack of safety awareness;
- unusual circumstances.

Some of these factors apply to the child from a 'good' home as well as to the child from a deprived background.

Points for discussion

- Are childhood accidents preventable given the inherent nature of children?

- Are accidents always due to lack of adult supervision?
- What other factors contribute to childhood accidents?

In a survey undertaken by the British Paediatric Association, the British Association of Paediatric Surgeons and the Casualty Surgeons Association in 1987, it was found that children comprise one-quarter of all patients attending Accident and Emergency departments annually.

The same study has shown that 20–25% of the child population will attend A and E departments annually, approximately 2–2.5 million children.

Point for discussion

- Whose responsibility is it to create a safe environment for the child?

The purpose of this chapter is to examine the care of the child and his or her family or carers in A and E departments. To do this a number of issues require exploration as outlined in the introduction. These issues include the physical and emotional needs of the child and his or her carers, the reasons why children are brought to A and E departments, parental involvement in care and the development of philosophies for the continuing care of the child in A and E. Other issues will be examined such as the death of a child, non-accidental injury, the Children Act 1989 and community liaison.

THE CHILD: EMOTIONAL AND PHYSICAL NEEDS

All children are unique, developing individuals. Their development includes physical, emotional, psychological and social elements (RCN, 1990) and they are totally dependent upon parents or familiar carers for security and love.

The care of the child in an A and E department must be based on the philosophy and the practice of family centred care. Such care is influenced by two separate disciplines (Webb and Cleaver, 1991): firstly the discipline of A and E, dominated by the needs of patients requiring urgent medical attention, and secondly the paediatric nurse's discipline which is committed to the ethos of family centred care (Toohey and Field, 1985). The National Association for the Welfare of Children and Young People in Hospital (1984) have published guidelines which have as their main aim the recognition of the best practice in dealing with children and their families. These guidelines are based on the conviction that the greatest harm to children in hospital is occasioned by separation from their mother (Shelley, 1991). Therefore a philosophy of care of the child in A and E will contain both physical, psychological and social elements and will plan for the involvement of the family as a unit. Any documentation should reflect this.

Just as children are susceptible to accidents, they are also prone to illness. Their immune systems are immature and extremes of heat, fluid and electrolyte loss, infection and tissue injury are not well tolerated by children (Webb and Cleaver, 1991).

Points for discussion

● Discuss the physiological response of the child to sudden illness.

● Discuss ways in which parents or carers could become involved in their child's care in A and E.

For a child, a visit to an A and E department can be a frightening experience. The child may never have been in hospital before; everything is strange and new . . . the atmosphere, the smells, the sounds of distress from adults and other children can reach nightmare proportions (Burton, 1993a). A child will cling to his or her mother or father with tenacity. In familiarity there is security. Even the child

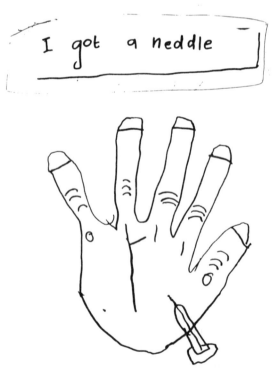

Figure 10.1 'I got a neddle.'

who has been abused physically, sexually or emotionally will cling to his abusers rather than trust a safe stranger (RCN, 1990). When all this emotional upset is allied to a physical reason for attendance it is easy to understand the vulnerability and fear.

If children are being seen in an adult A and E department it is important that their waiting area is separate from that of adults. They should be shielded from the sights and sounds of adults requiring treatment and from the sights, sounds and smells of intoxicated and/or aggressive adults (RCN, 1990).

The joint working party of the RCN's A and E Forum and Paediatric Society (RCN, 1990) found that the care children receive in A and E departments may not always be conducive to their physical and emotional well-being.

Points for discussion

● Discuss the emotional response of a child when in A and E.

● Why should a child cling to his or her abusers when a 'safe' nurse is available?

● How can children attending A and E departments be shielded from the sights and sounds of distressed adults?

● In what ways could the care children receive in A and E be harmful to their physical and emotional well-being?

If children are emotionally mishandled in the A and E department and are not treated with a sensitive awareness of their needs, a visit to A and E may cause psychological scars which may be with them for a long time (Burton, 1993a).

Every aspect of their care must be seen through the eyes of a child and planned accordingly. It helps if the environment is child orientated. Equipment such as chairs and tables should be childsized, walls painted with bright murals depicting favourite and familiar characters, beloved of children. Posters and children's own paintings and drawings make an area less threatening and give the child an opportunity to influence the environment with minimal expenditure (RCN, 1990).

Points for discussion

● Discuss how the environment of A and E could be made more child orientated.

● Should children have separate waiting areas in an adult A an E department?

Any area which is designated for the use of children should be

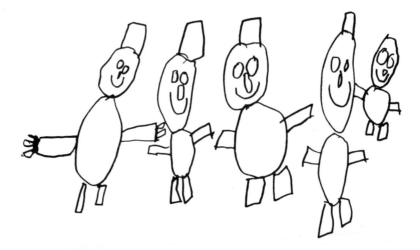

Figure 10.2 Staff seen through the eyes of a child.

adequately supplied with toys which are safe, easily cleaned and indestructible. Children learn through play and play is now recognized as an essential part of normal development. Play is also a useful tool to educate and to inform.

Some A and E departments now have a play specialist as part of their team. Toys must be chosen carefully and with safety in mind. It is important, therefore, that toys should be larger than those which could be ingested or inhaled. If soft toys are provided they should be easily washed. Dolls and teddies could be used to demonstrate treatments and procedures.

Children learn to play and they learn through play. In play they imitate real situations. Wordsworth (1960) in his poem 'Intimations of Immortality' describes it thus: 'as if their whole vocation were endless imitation'.

Points for discussion

- Discuss what toys would be suitable for use in the play area of an A and E department.

- How can a child's inherent propensity for play be channelled into a learning process?

- Should the play specialist attend staff meetings in the A and E department?

Nurses and medical staff need to take time to build up a rapport with the child. Children must not be ignored but should be included in the conversation, perhaps by talking about what they are wearing or about a toy they may have with them.

It is one of the most rewarding aspects of the paediatric nurse's work to gain the trust and confidence of the child. Children have inarticulated needs and nurses need to recognize that a silent withdrawn child is shouting as loudly as the child who is screaming and struggling (RCN, 1990).

In 1991 an article was published in the *Americn Journal of Emergency Nursing* called 'How to deal with children in the emergency department'. Its author, Donna Thomas (1991), makes the following recommendations:

- Gain the child's confidence;
- Treat the child firmly but kindly;
- Give the child your approval and smiles;
- Never be impatient or lose your temper;
- Make haste slowly;
- Tell the child now brave he/she was.

Parents should be encouraged to stay with their child at all times except perhaps in an emergency situation, for examle where resuscitation is being carried out. Parents should be included in the nurse's conversation with the child and an attempt made to gain their cooperation and their trust. They may be trying to cope with feelings of guilt, blaming themselves for the accident. This may not be articulated but sensed by the staff.

Points for discussion

- Should parents be allowed in the resuscitation room if they wish?

- Would you describe a silent child as a 'good' child and a noisy, vociferous child as a 'bad' child?

- How would you cope with a mother who was blaming herself for the child's accident?

If at all possible the child should be allowed to remain on the parent's knee and they can be encouraged to help the child undress or, if the child is too young, to do it for them.

Children will cling to their clothes with determination, seeing them as their link with security and familiarity (Burton, 1993a). Children need privacy as much as adults and a child's modesty and dignity should always be protected.

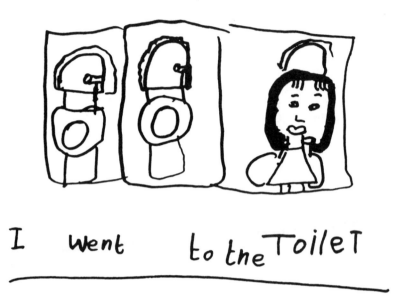

I went to the Toilet

Figure 10.3 'I went to the toilet.'

MANPOWER AND TRIAGE

In the Department of Health's *Guidelines for the Welfare of Children and Young People in Hospital* (1991), the following recommendation is made: 'Medical and nursing staff trained and experienced in the care of children must be available at all times'. The RCN (1990) recommends that each A and E department should attempt to recruit a registered sick children's nurse (RSCN) to its staff. The RSCN would act as an advocate for the children as a group and as a facilitator for other staff. RSCN cover for 24 hours per day is vital but not always possible. The RCN also recommends that 'each A and E department should have one RSCN on its staff who is qualified or experienced in A and E nursing'.

A RSCN, who has been specially trained in the care of children, will understand the special needs of the child and family. The RSCN will understand what is normal in a child's development and recognize the alteration in physiology and the response of a child to illness or injury. Included within this recognition and understanding are the physiological effects of injury, sickness and hospitalization (RCN, 1990).

A child's first contact with the A and E department will usually be at the reception desk. Here personal details are recorded and the child will be given relevant documentation. The documentation will vary from hospital to hospital. The RCN (1990) recommends that A and E records should be computerized, thus facilitating easy retrieval and quantification of attendances at a department. Many A and E departments are moving over to such systems. Information available on the documentation should include:

- name
- address
- age
- general practitioner's name and address
- school
- health visitor
- a record of previous visits.

Many A and E departments are now practising triage. Triage is defined as 'the assignment of degrees of urgency to decide on order of treatment, wounds, illnesses, etcetera' (*Concise Oxford Dictionary*, 1990). Ideally every child should be seen by the triage nurse immediately following arrival in the department.

Triage is particularly important where children are concerned because of their physiological vulnerability to rapid deterioration in their condition. The triage nurse should be experienced and able to make a knowledgeable assessment and to prioritize safely.

The triage nurse, while speaking to the child and parents, should be observing, assessing and, while focusing on the present injury and its requisite treatment, should be taking into account the wider social and environmental issues involved (Webb and Cleaver, 1991). The triage nurse should be a RSCN if he or she is dealing with children in an A and E department.

Studies concerning triage make no reference to prioritizing children (Webb and Cleaver, 1991). Some A and E departments do prioritize children but this may not always be possible.

Points for discussion

- Should children always be given priority in A and E departments?

- Why is it so important for each child to be seen by a RSCN?

- Why is it necessary to record the name of the child's school on the documentation?

- What is the most important function of the triage nurse?

The DoH *Guidelines* (1991) recommend that A and E departments should have 'effective procedures to prioritize waiting children and ensure that they are seen promptly'.

As well as medical and nursing staff, many other disciplines are involved in the workings of A and E departments. These include:

- The health visitor, who may have a valuable follow-up role. The health visitor can reinforce advice given to parents in the department at home.
- The play specialist. Some paediatric A and E departments have appointed play specialists.
- The social worker is closely involved with the A and E department team. The medical social worker has a key role in coordinating the investigation of suspected child abuse (RCN, 1990).
- The radiographer. Many children attending A and E because of illness or injury will require an X-ray.
- The dietitian. Often children are brought to A and E, for example, complaining of abdominal pain and this is found to be due to constipation or a mother may be having problems with her baby who is vomiting. The dietitian is available for advice.
- The physiotherapist. Occasionally a child may be referred to the physiotherapist directly from A and E, for example, following an injury or an illness such as a chest infection.

This list is not fully comprehensive; there may be other sources of referral which are part of the child's continuing care in A and E such as the clinical psychologist or the various outpatient departments.

REASONS FOR COMING TO ACCIDENT AND EMERGENCY

Many parents attending A and E departments with children are substituting their visit for a family doctor consultation. These children have been described as 'inappropriate attenders'.

'Inappropriate attenders' were viewed as 'those who did not fit into an accident or emergency category and should have, more appropriately, attended their own general practitioner for treatment' (Bolton and Storrie, 1991). It is not the role of the nurse to judge the legitimacy of a patient's or a parent's visit to the department.

The reasons children are brought to A and E are as varied as the personalities of the children themselves.

In a retrospective study of the year 1988 carried out in the A and E department of the Queen's Medical Centre, Nottingham, one-third of inappropriate attenders were parents whose children were under one year old. Over half were under three years of age. Problems relating to the digestive and the respiratory tract were most common (Bolton and Storrie, 1991).

In a similar study carried out in the A and E department of the Royal Belfast Hospital for Sick Children (Burton, 1989), in one

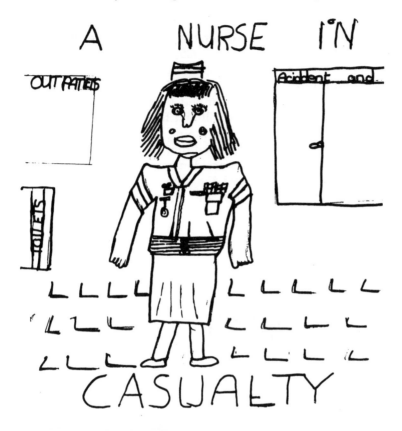

Figure 10.4 'A nurse in casualty.'

24-hour period 108 children were seen. They were classified as follows:

- Medical – 33 (30%)
- Surgical – 16 (15%)
- Accidents – 20 (19%)
- Emergencies – 3 (3%)
- Other reasons – 36 (33%).

Other reasons for attendance included ENT, dermatology, orthopaedic and social problems. This was a winter month survey (October–March) and experience shows that the pattern changes completely during the summer months.

Many attendances were shown to be associated with the need for reassurance and advice.

Many children cannot be classified as 'inappropriate attenders' and are in A and E because of trauma. At all ages during childhood, road traffic accidents are the leading cause of death (Alpar and Owen, 1988).

The environment poses many hazards to children and many come to grief while developing an understanding and respect for the world around them (Alpar and Owen, 1988).

In Belfast a major project is being carried out by the North and West Belfast Community Unit and the Child Accident Prevention Trust (McMillan and Mercer, 1992) funded by the Making Belfast Work Initiative. The project, which will last for three years, will look at childhood accidents in total, their timing and type and the conditions under which they occur. It is hoped that the study will have a major impact upon the reduction of accidents, not only in N. Ireland but in the remainder of the United Kingdom. In March 1992 an interim analysis was made (McMillan and Mercer, 1992). The following information emerged:

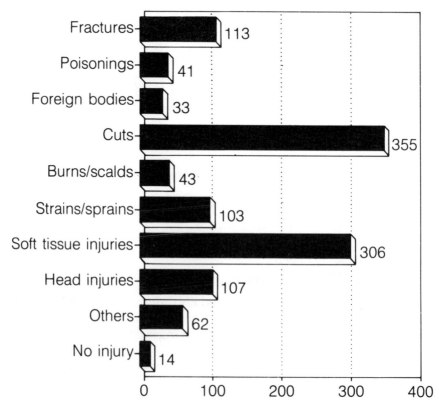

Figure 10.5 Types of injuries sustained (North and West Belfast Community Unit and the Child Accident Prevention Trust, 1992).

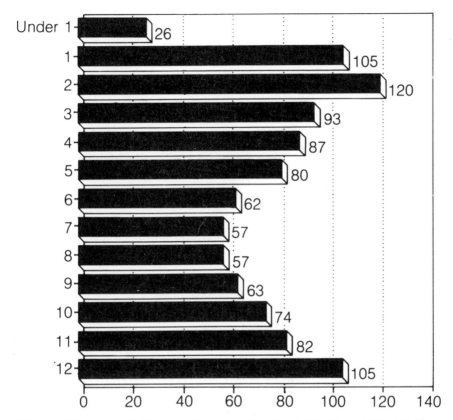

Figure 10.6 Age of children at the time of accident (North and West Belfast Community Unit and the Child Accident Prevention Trust, 1992).

- Total number in sample – 1074 children
- Lacerations – 355
- Soft tissue injuries – 306
- Fractures – 113
- Head injuries – 107
- Others – 62
- Burns/scalds – 43
- Poisoning – 41
- Foreign bodies – 33
- No injury – 14

The majority of children were in the 0–5 year group and in the 12-year-old group. Most children were injured in their own home; Tuesday and Sunday were the busiest days. The vast majority of injuries were classified as minor, that is, not life-threatening or requiring hospitalization. The project is being carried out with the cooperation of the A and E departments of the Royal Belfast Hospital for Sick Children and the Mater Infirmorum Hospital, Belfast.

Points for discussion

- Why do many parents substitute a visit to A and E for a visit to their general practitioner?

- Who should decide whether a child's attendance at A and E is appropriate or not?

- Should children with apparently trivial injuries ever be refused treatment?

- How can nurses working in A and E departments meet the parents' need for reassurance and advice?

- Discuss why childhood accidents are most common in the 1–5-year-old age group (see Fig. 10.6).

- Why should the pattern of childhood accidents peak again at 12 years of age (see Fig. 10.6)?

STANDARDS FOR CHILDREN IN THE ACCIDENT AND EMERGENCY DEPARTMENT

A standard is defined by the *Concise Oxford Dictionary* (1990) in several ways. The definitions most applicable to nursing practice are these:

- An object or quality or measure serving as a basis or example or principle to which others conform or should conform;
- the degree of excellence required for a specific purpose;
- a thing recognized as a model for imitation.

Therefore standards are a basis for nursing children in A and E. They are examples of good practice and incorporate principles and philosophies which are excellent in theory and practice and have as their model for imitation the well-being of the child and family. The DoH (1991) and other professional bodies have provided recommendations for child care. In 1990 the RCN A and E Forum and the Society of Paediatric Nursing produced an excellent booklet called *Nursing Children in the Accident and Emergency Department*.

On 14 October 1991 the Children Act 1989 became law. Designed to promote the interests of all children, the Act represents the most fundamental reform of legislation affecting children to occur this century. It sets standards for the way we as a society want to see our children brought up and protected (RCN, 1990). The Children Act will be discussed on page 199.

Many A and E departments have been involved in the definition of their own standards, within the broader guidelines of these documents. Standards are inherent in our practice, both personally and professionally. It is important that every member of the A and E team becomes involved in the setting of department standards for the continuing care of the child and family. The Royal College of Nursing's A and E Forum and Society of Paediatric Nursing (1990) suggest that 'The standard of care given to the patient is to a great extent dependent upon the staff available to deliver the care'. This is where the RSCN may be used as a resource and as an advocate for the child and family. The RSCN should be fully involved in the setting and monitoring of standards. Standards should be realistic and achievable.

All standards for children in A and E should reflect the child's right to be viewed as an individual, in the context of his family of which he is an integral member and from which he derives emotional and physical support (RCN, 1990). This chapter has already discussed the physical and psychological needs of the child. Children have a great fear of the unknown and of separation from their parents. They also fear pain and the unspoken threat of painful procedures. Parents should always be encouraged to stay with their child; they can assist by holding the child as certain procedures are carried out, for example venepuncture or X-ray.

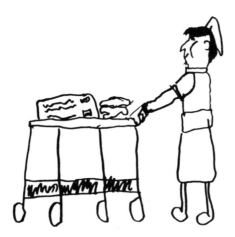

Figure 10.7 The unspoken threat of further painful procedures.

The DoH (1991) recommends that 'parents should be able to give continuous love and support to their child and especially be together with their child at the most stressful time ...'.

Points for discussion

● Discuss the role of the RSCN when setting standards for the care of the child and family in A and E.

● Discuss ways of auditing practice in A and E.

● How can consumer satisfaction be measured when the patient is a child?

● What is meant by this statement: 'Standards should be realistic and achievable'?

AUDITING PRACTICE IN ACCIDENT AND EMERGENCY

Many A and E departments are setting their own standards and auditing their practice. A standard is simply a defined degree of excellence required for a particular purpose and before the quality can be measured there needs to be a basic (example) principle against which the measurement can be taken. The *Accident and Emergency Monitor* (Dutton *et al.*, 1991) is a quality assurance tool designed for use in A and E. It provides a series of master checklists of observable, quality related criteria by which nurses can assess the quality of care. It also contains a junior supplement. Included with the *Monitor* is a patient satisfaction questionnaire but many A and E departments are designing their own. Where children are concerned it will be a parent satisfaction questionnaire except where the child is of an age to answer personally.

The parents' views reflect those of the child and their perceptions of care are a valuable indicator to the quality of the A and E service. Any deficiencies can be identified and action taken to correct them. Only by listening to the patients can we hope to improve care. Only when practitioners identify a personal commitment to changing practice and recognize the role parents' views might have in identifying where changes are required will paediatric units become fully self-evaluating (Ball *et al.*, 1988).

By trying to assess parental satisfaction nurses are meeting the standard which encapsulates the philosophy of partnership with the family in caring for the child.

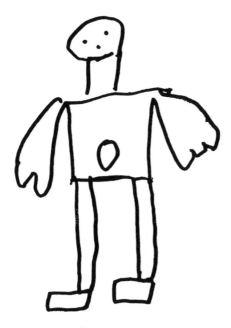

Figure 10.8 The parents' views reflect those of the child.

Points for discussion

- Who should be involved in setting standards in A and E?

- How can these standards be monitored?

- What tools might be used to measure parent satisfaction with A and E services?

- What steps could be taken to correct any deficiencies identified by the audit process?

THE CHILDREN ACT 1989

The Royal College of Nursing in conjunction with the Department of Health (1992) have produced a very useful booklet called *The Children Act (1989) – What Every Nurse, Health Visitor and Midwife Needs to Know*. It clearly sets out the main principles of the Act and defines the implications of the Act for district health authorities, NHS trusts and family health service authorities. The booklet describes the implications for practitioners and defines a child in need as follows.

1. He is unlikely to achieve or maintain, or have the opportunity of achieving or maintaining, a reasonable standard of health or development without the provision for him of services by a local authority.
2. His health or development is likely to be significantly impaired or further impaired without the provision for him of such services.
3. He is disabled.

Because A and E nurses are often the first people to identify problems within the child or within the family unit such as a poor standard of health or that the child's development is behind, the Children Act 1989 has particular relevance for them. The nurse in A and E may be the first to notice, for example, that the child is dirty and/or uncared for, that there are signs of suspected child abuse, physical, sexual or emotional.

The RCN/DoH (1992) booklet states that:

> Any nurse who comes into contact with children may be the first person to alert others, in particular paediatric nurses, nurses working in A and E departments, psychiatric nurses, mental handicap nurses and practice nurses, who will need to have an agreed practice protocol.

The Children Act 1989 is designed to promote the interests of all children. The Act specifies that the welfare of children is the paramount consideration. It aims to strike a balance between family autonomy and the rights of children.

Each health authority in the UK will have its own policy on dealing with children who are suspected of having been abused or neglected. Each A and E department should be familar with this policy and have a copy of procedures to be carried out.

A and E nurses need to familiarize themselves with court orders which have particular relevance to practitioners. These orders include the following.

Care order

Made if the court decides a child is suffering or likely to suffer significant harm through lack of adequate parental care or control (RCN/DoH, 1992).

The A and E nurse may be the first person to notice that a child is having repeated accidents, for example, or seems to be unsupervised by an adult. A care order places the child in the care of the local authority who then share responsibility with the parents.

Supervision order

Made if the court decides that the local authority should keep a close eye on the child and give guidance (RCN/DoH, 1992).

Child assessment order

This is a completely new order which addresses those situations where there is reasonable cause to suspect that a child is suffering significant harm but is not at immediate risk.

If the applicant believes that an assessment is required and the parents are unwilling to cooperate, a representative from the local authority or the National Society for the Prevention of Cruelty to Children (NSPCC) may apply.

Emergency protection order (EPO)

Replaces the place of safety order and is only made in extremely urgent cases when the child's safety is immediately threatened. This order may be made for a maximum of eight days with one possible extension of seven days. Any person may apply for this order but it is usually the local authority or the NSPCC. The applicant is given parental responsibility for the child only insofar as it is necessary in order to safeguard and promote the welfare of the child (RCN/DoH, 1992).

The difference between a care order and an emergency protection order is that in the care order the parents have equal responsibility with the local authority and with the EPO the applicant has total responsibility.

Points for discussion

- The Children Act 1989 – discuss its implications for A and E nursing.
- Why is it so important for every A and E department to have its own practice protocol?

NON-ACCIDENTAL INJURY

Child abuse is not new (Helfer and Helfer, 1980). It has existed for centuries with varying degrees of acceptance by society. In the 20th century, when the standard of child care has never been higher, it is difficult to realize that child abuse has become a major social problem (Helfer and Helfer, 1980). This includes physical, sexual and emotional abuse. Previously the physical and emotional well-being of a child was left to his parents (Radbill, 1980). This was fine if the child was cared for physically and loved and supported by his or her carers both psychologically and emotionally. In Dickensian England (1812–1870) the status of the child in society was low and literature abounded with stories of physical and emotional neglect of children.

Nurses working in A and E departments must be aware of abuse's many faces. Physical and/or sexual abuse may be more easy to detect than emotional abuse. Physical abuse may range from bruising to the death of a child.

Physical, emotional or sexual abuse may exist as single entities but often occur in combination (Radbill, 1980).

There is a need for nurses to develop a 'listening ear', to recognize the *cri de coeur*. Occasionally a parent may confide in the nurse that they are afraid of what they might do to their child. This should never be ignored. Again, the parent who continually brings their child to A and E with seemingly trivial injuries may be saying the same thing. The mother may say 'He is always crying or always vomiting' and no cause can be found. In the majority of situations abuse is seldom mentioned and nurses must develop skills which enable them to build up a picture of parents, of the child and of the events surrounding the injury. A balance needs to be struck between ensuring the safety and well-being of the child and safeguarding the parents who may well be entirely innocent. The parents may not be the abusers. Physical signs such as bruising may turn out to be due to an illness.

The nurse working in A and E departments and dealing with parents and children needs to:

- develop listening skills;
- develop an informed awareness of the signs of potential abuse;
- use skilled, experienced observation;
- have a knowledge of correct action and use of multidisciplinary resources.

It must be remembered that two-thirds of all **physically** abused children are under three years of age because they are defenceless, demanding and non-verbal. Child abuse is only the symptom, seen when a family's interactional system has broken down (Helfer and Helfer, 1980).

> The constant, uncontrollable crying of a baby may trigger off child abuse in a susceptible parent.
>
> (*Steele, 1980*)

Parents and/or carers who abuse their children may be immature and dependent. They often have poor impulse control and a low tolerance of frustration (Helfer and Helfer, 1980).

Nurses working in A and E need to be aware and sensitive to the unarticulated needs of children and their families; they should be knowledgeable and familiar with both local and national policies and procedures. Often child abuse is not explicit but is intuitively perceived by an experienced person.

Points for discussion

● Discuss the role of the nurse in the early detection of child abuse in A and E.

● How can nurses recognize a *cri de coeur* from a parent?

● How important is it to have a local policy for dealing with children who are suspected of having been abused?

THE DEATH OF A CHILD

It is inevitable that nurses working in the emergency situation will eventually be faced with the death of a child.

All staff faced with the death of a child may have feelings of inadequacy and question inwardly how they can ease the pain of bereavement or bring comfort to a grieving family.

When a severely injured child is brought into the department and dies or when a baby is carried in who is a victim of sudden infant death, one nurse should be assigned to stay with the parents and relatives at all times. This nurse will be responsible for keeping the family informed of what is happening, helping them to contact friends or their minister of religion (Burton, 1993a). Practical measures, such as having any other children looked after, need to be addressed. It is important that the same nurse remains with the family when the death of their child is confirmed.

In every A and E department there should be a room where bereaved parents and/or siblings can begin the grieving process in private. It is better if this room is sited somewhere away from the clinical area, from the sights and sounds of other children and their parents. If at all possible the mother and father or others of their choice should be allowed to hold their little one for as long as they want to. Their religious and cultural beliefs must be respected.

The DoH (1991) specify the following standard:

Parents are given the privacy to grieve alone in a quiet room, set aside for this purpose, with the body of their child if they so wish.

Parents will want to talk and usually ask many questions. They may want to tell the nurse, over and over again, of their baby or child's last hours. They may be very articulate and angry or they may be shocked and withdrawn. However they demonstrate their grief, the nurse should be ready to listen, to answer questions and to give knowledgeable professional advice.

Every A and E department will have its own policies and procedures to follow in these circumstances. If staff are familiar with them and have clear written guidelines to follow, they will feel more confident about coping with the parents.

Many departments have bereavement packs for the parents of victims of sudden infant death. This may contain a polaroid photograph of the baby, a lock of hair, the imprint of their baby's foot as well as information and support groups such as the Foundation for the Study of Sudden Infant Death (1992). A relative or friend can be given written instructions about the removal of the body, the funeral arrangements and the post mortem.

Nurses themselves, especially junior staff, should receive counselling and support from their more senior colleagues. They should be encouraged to talk about how they felt and how they coped in a situation which is traumatic for all.

If nurses are familar with the practicalities and knowledgeable about correct procedure, they can demonstrate with confidence a philosophy of care which is sensitive to the needs of families who grieve.

Points for discussion

● Nurses should never allow parents to see that they are upset when a child dies. Discuss this statement.

● Discuss the role of voluntary agencies to help when parents are bereaved.

● How can nurses help each other in this situation?

SOME THOUGHTS ABOUT RESEARCH

Increasingly nurses are learning to make their practice research based. Research is 'an endeavour to discover new or collate old facts by the scientific study of a subject or by a course of critical investigation' (*Concise Oxford Dictionary*, 1990). A and E nurses are uniquely placed to discover new facts and to collate old facts. There is a wealth of information available. Through research methods nurses can observe the pattern of certain accidents and, for example, the age group most at risk (see Figs 10.5 and 10.6).

Nurses in the A and E department of the Royal Belfast Hospital for Sick Children, concerned about the number of children being admitted having taken tablets or other poisons, carried out a survey over a period of one year. Results indicated that particular concerns may be justified. In cooperation with other agencies such as the Royal Society for the Prevention of Accidents, the Home Accident Prevention Council and the media, an attempt was made to reach the public with the message of the seriousness of the problem (Burton, 1993b). The results of the survey were published in the local paper. Nurses who took part in the survey were interviewed on Radio Ulster.

The author was asked to speak to various mother and toddler groups. A leaflet, warning of the dangers, is being published in conjunction with the Royal Belfast Hospital for Sick Children and the Regional Drugs and Poisons Information Service (1993).

This study is cited to illustrate how research can be used by nurses in the clinical situation to improve the quality of care given to their young patients. Research challenges traditional practice, it threatens cherished theories, it stirs us to question and to evaluate in a systematic and thorough way.

Not all nurses can be researchers but all nurses can be readers and evaluators of other people's research and can decide on possible implications for their practice. Research awareness should be fostered in paediatric A and E departments and research interest and skills identified and developed. Opportunities for further education and training should be given to nurses in A and E who wish to develop their research interest and skills.

Points for discussion

● How can research improve the care of the child and family in A and E?

● Who should be carrying out the research in nursing?

● How can nurses improve their research skills?

THE WELL TEDDY CLINIC

Large numbers of children attend A and E departments each year. For many children it is their first experience of being in hospital. The environment is strange, the smells, the noise, the uniforms are alarming (RCN, 1990).

Children are always vulnerable but even more if they are sick or injured. It is difficult to gain their trust and remove their fear. They feel threatened, out of control and experience stress.

Play therapy, in all its forms, can help alleviate such stress and facilitate a smoother adjustment to the new and potentially frightening

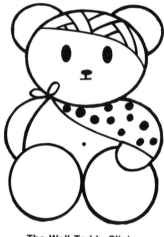

The Well Teddy Clinic

Figure 10.9 The Well Teddy clinic.

surroundings (Doverty, 1992). In the Royal Belfast Hospital for Sick Children, a 'Well Teddy clinic' is held regularly. This gives an opportunity for **well** children to come into the hospital environment, to handle non-injurious hospital equipment, for example auriscopes and stethoscopes, to dress up in real uniforms, play with hospital orientated toys and generally become familiar with many of the activities they may see in A and E. All activities are centred on their teddy bear and this means the children feel less threatened (Golden, 1990).

Staff in the Flint Osteopathic Hospital identified a need to 'create a positive image of the hospital as a caring, friendly institution and to decrease children's levels of unfamiliarity and anxiety' (Golden, 1990). Children in local playgroups are invited to bring Teddy for a check-up. Teddy is subjected to an examination similar to the one the child might receive in A and E. The clinic even has a triage nurse.

The clinic is a service to potential patients, their parents and the community (Burton, 1991). The Well Teddy clinic sounds like fun but it all requires time, dedication and meticulous planning. It has implication for resources both in manpower and financial terms.

Points for discussion

- Does the end justify the means?
- Should nurses be concentrating on the needs of sick children and not on the education of well children?

● What are the advantages of introducing children to the hospital environment when they are well?

POSSIBLE OUTCOMES OF A CHILD'S VISIT TO A AND E

When a child is brought to an emergency department there are four possible outcomes:

1. discharge home;
2. admission;
3. transfer to another hospital;
4. referral to another source.

Discharge home is, of course, the desired outcome by A and E staff (Burton, 1993a).

The DoH (1991) recommend that children shall be admitted to hospital only if the care they require cannot be equally provided at home or on a day basis. Discharge home often involves liaison with community personnel such as the general practitioner, the health visitor and the district nurse.

The success of discharge home depends on good communication, both verbal and written, so that parents understand clearly all advice and instruction. Information and advice should be both verbal and written. Printed leaflets should be available on such subjects as:

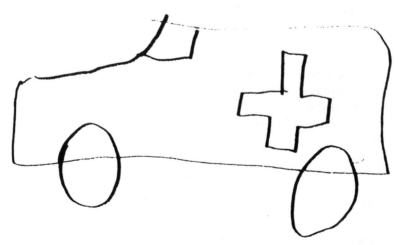

Figure 10.10 Transfer to another hospital.

- head injury;
- care of plaster of Paris;
- febrile convulsions;
- control of pyrexia;
- management of diarrhoea and vomiting.

These help the family to continue care at home. Leaflets containing instructions should be printed in languages other than English.

In conjunction with the information given to parents, information can also be given to children in the form of a story book or colouring book. The books, though fun, should also contain an educational message for the child.

Parents should be reassured that they can phone the A and E department any time for advice.

Admission

When the decision is taken to admit a child to the ward, old fears, temporarily allayed, may cause the child to become very agitated. They will begin to see their worst fears realized ... the fear of separation, the fear of the unknown (RCN, 1990). They will sense parental anxiety also and may imitate fears.

Distress will be lessened if the same nurse is responsible for their care from the moment they come into the unit until the moment the child is handed over to the ward staff. This nurse will already have established a rapport with the child and parents and should be involved in the preparation of the child for admission.

A favourite toy can be admitted with the child and have an identity armband also.

The nurse should explain, perhaps with the help of pictures, what the ward will be like and why the child has to be admitted. The child should be assured by 'their' nurse that Mummy and/or Daddy can stay.

This same nurse will be responsible for seeing that the appropriate documentation is complete, for informing the ward staff what is already known about the child, their condition and any treatment they may have had. The parents will need support and information also (Burton, 1993a).

Transfer to other hospitals

If a child requires transfer to another hospital, it may be for one of several reasons:

- The hospital may have no paediatric inpatient beds.
- The hospital may have filled its paediatric beds.

- The child may require specialized treatment, for example in a burns unit, or they may require isolation from other children because they are suffering from an infectious illness such as gastroenteritis.

The transfer of a child to another hospital is not an ideal situation as it involves further disruption to the child and family but unfortunately it is often necessary. The location of the receiving hospital may make it more difficult for parents to travel.

A joint statement from the British Paediatric Association, the British Association of Paediatric Surgeons and the Casualty Surgeons Association (1987) recommends that A and E departments where children are seen and children's departments should be on the same site and hospital and district planning should take account of this. When transfer must take place, it should be planned carefully to ensure the maximum welfare of the child, both physically and emotionally.

The joint working party of the Royal College of Nursing's A and E Forum and the Society of Paediatric Nursing (RCN, 1990) makes the following suggestions for a checklist:

- Have the parents and the child been told why transfer is necessary?
- Has the child received sufficient analgesia if necessary?
- Has there been sufficient interchange of information between the two hospitals?
- Is there a nurse or doctor available to accompany the child if necessary?
- Have the parents and child been introduced to the ambulance personnel?
- Is the child's condition stable?

Points for discussion

● How may the parents and the child be led to understand the need for transfer?

● How may the child be assured that Mummy and Daddy can go too?

● How may the child's condition be evaluated?

INFORMATION AND EDUCATION IN ACCIDENT AND EMERGENCY

Nurses working in A and E departments are uniquely placed to inform and educate. This is particularly true for RSCNs working in A and E. In their special role as the children's nurse they should be taking every opportunity to advise and teach. This is an essential part of nurses' professional responsibility to be both health educators and health promoters.

Advice may be given, quite informally, as the nurse establishes a relationship with the child and parents. There is often an opportunity to talk about accident prevention, for example the safe storage of drugs and poisons in the home. Parents very often come for reassurance and advice and this furnishes another opportunity for health promotion. Education should never be given to people in a scolding manner.

Educational videos can be shown in children's waiting areas on a variety of subjects:

- immunization status
- home safety
- road safety

Imaginative use of bright posters is another resource for teaching. These may be painted by the children themselves under the supervision of the play specialist. Local schools could become involved. Involving the children themselves creates more interest.

While listening, a nurse may detect the need for advice from the dietitian, for example, or from others. The triage nurse, while assessing the child, may identify lack of knowledge about proper diet or about which baby milks to use. Many children attend A and E departments every year with abdominal pain which is caused by constipation. This

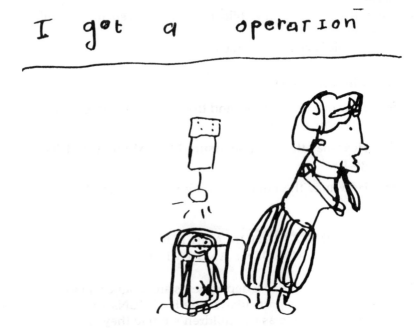

Figure 10.11 'I got a operation.'

often requires interventions which are distressing to the child such as the giving of suppositories or an enema. In such a situation nurses have an opportunity to talk about the part poor diet plays in the cause of constipation. 'Home made bread or brown bread is a most important article of diet for many patients. The use of aperients may be entirely superseded by it' (Nightingale, quoted in Baley, 1991).

The nurse will be able to talk with the mother or father about why the child is not immunized, if applicable.

It is debatable just how much parents retain in the stress of a visit to an A and E department; however, the opportunity must be taken and followed up by appropriate liaison with other disciplines where necessary. Verbal advice and teaching should be reinforced by giving written advice.

LIAISON WITH THE COMMUNITY

Liaison with the community and primary health care team will provide a more holistic approach to care and enhance communication between the disciplines providing care to the child and his family.

(RCN, 1990)

As the desired outcome for children attending A and E is discharge home (RCN, 1990), the importance of adequate communication with community personnel cannot be overemphasized. Children are especially vulnerable to any shortcomings in hospital discharge arrangements, particularly those who are at risk of abuse, who have long term disabilities or whose parents seem unwilling to care for them (DoH, 1991).

The liaison health visitor has an important role to play, with regular contact with the family in their home. The A and E nurse has only a short contact with the child and family but the liaison health visitor can follow up attenders and give advice on accident prevention in the home. The health visitor may be the person to identify any problems in the home situation.

The medical social worker has a key role to play in coordinating the investigation of suspected cases of child abuse and can deal with social problems which arise and perhaps domestic problems also.

Other liaison personnel who may be involved with the care of the child are:

- the district nurse
- the school nurse
- the practice nurse

Good quality discharge procedure contains the following elements:

- continuing support for the family;
- social support;
- notification to the general practitioner;
- notification to the health visitor;
- transport arrangements if necessary;
- provision of necessary equipment, dressings or medicines with instructions for their use;
- notification to the parents of arrangements for an outpatient attendance.

These recommendations are taken from the DoH *Guidelines* (1991).

Points for discussion

- What are the implications for the use/non-use of the DoH *Guidelines* (1991) in A and E?

- Discuss how hospital and community personnel can work together to provide continuing support for the child and family.

CONCLUSION

Children are unique, developing individuals with very special needs and although it is often a physical condition which brings them to A and E, their psychological, emotional and social needs must be met also. This includes their family's need. The child's physical needs are the most demanding in an A and E situation but the child's care must be planned with these other needs in view. Children are susceptible

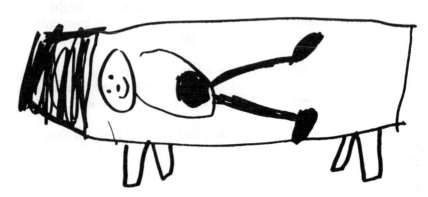

Figure 10.12 Unique, developing individuals.

to injury, accidental or otherwise, they deteriorate quickly and may recover just as quickly.

They should be assessed within the context of their own family. If a child is unaccompanied a full assessment should be made of both the presenting problem and the reasons for the child being unaccompanied. The nurse, at this stage, should decide whether parental consent is required (RCN, 1990).

Children need the care of specially trained staff (RSCNs). The children's waiting area should be separate from that of the adults and should be child orientated. All equipment including resuscitation equipment should be childsized. A chart giving paediatric drug doses should be displayed in the resuscitation room.

Parents must be allowed to stay with their children at all times.

Protocols should be developed for dealing with non-accidental injury or sudden infant death.

A and E departments, in developing their philosophy of care for children, need to consider all these elements.

Nursing children in A and E requires special skills, not only clinical skills but skills in communicating and in understanding. Children and their families attending A and E deserve excellence in both philosophical concept and in practice. This is achieved through training and experience and a commitment to research based practice.

REFERENCES

Alpar, E.K. and Owen, R. (1988) *Paediatric Trauma*, 1st edn, Castle House Publications, Tunbridge Wells, Kent.

Baley, M (ed.) (1991) *As Miss Nightingale Said*, Scutari Press, Harrow, Middlesex.

Ball, M., Glasper, A. and Yerrell, P. (1988) How well do we perform? Parents' perceptions of paediatric care. Quality assurance in Paediatrics. *Professional Nurse*, 4(3), 115–18.

Bolton, K. and Storrie, C. (1991) Inappropriate attenders at A and E – Accident and Emergency. *Paediatric Nursing*, 3(2), 22–3.

British Paediatric Association/Association of Paediatric Surgeons/Casualty Surgeons Association (1987) Joint Statement on Children's Attendances at A/E Departments, British Paediatric Association, London, p. 42.

Burton, R. (1989) Shifting horizons – parents' perceptions of a paediatric A and E department. *Paediatric Nursing*, 1(8), 19–20.

Burton, R. (1991) Me and my teddy bear. *Nursing Standard*, 5(38), 20–1.

Burton, R. (1993a) The child in A and E: a philosophy of care, in *Advances in Child Health Nursing*, (eds E.A. Glasper and A. Turcher), Scutari Press, London.

Burton, R. (1993b) Eat, drink and be dead – a study of accidental ingestion of poisons in young children. *Accident and Emergency Nursing*, 1, 14–19.

Chesterfield, The Earl of (1979) *Oxford Dictionary of Quotations*, 3rd edn, Oxford University Press, New York, p. 145.

Concise Oxford Dictionary of Current English (1990) 8th edn, Clarendon Press, Oxford.

Department of Health (1991) *Guidelines for the Welfare of Children and Young People in Hospital*, HMSO, London.

Doverty, N. (1992) Therapeutic use of play in hospital. *British Journal of Nursing*, 1(2), 79–81.

Dutton, J., Grylls, L. and Goldstone, L. (1991) *Accident and Emergency Monitor*, Gale Centre Publications, Loughton, Essex.

Foundation for the Study of Sudden Infant Deaths (1992) *Sudden Infant Death*, FSSID, London.

Golden, I.J. (1990) Teddy bear clinic. *Journal of Emergency Nursing*, 16(5), 357.

Graydon, R. (1989) *Basic Principles of Child Accident Prevention*, Child Accident Prevention Trust, London.

Helfer, E.H. and Helfer, R.E. (1980) Communicating in the therapeutic relationship, in *The Battered Child*, (eds C.H. Kempe and R.E. Helfer), University of Chicago Press, Chicago.

McMillan, A. and Mercer, R. (1992) Child Accident Prevention Trust Project, unpublished interim report.

National Association for the Welfare of Children in Hospital (1984) *NAWCH Charter*, NAWCH, London.

Radbill, S.X. (1980) Children in a world of violence – a history of child abuse, in *The Battered Child*, (eds C.H. Kempe and R.E. Helfer), University of Chicago Press, Chicago.

Royal Belfast Hospital for Sick Children/NI Regional Drugs & Poisons Information Service (1993) *Deadly Deception*, leaflet on accidental ingestion of poisons, EHSSB, Belfast.

Royal College of Nursing A/E Forum/Society of Paediatric Nursing (1990) *Nursing Children in the Accident and Emergency Departments*, RCN, London.

Royal College of Nursing/Department of Health (1992) *What Every Nurse, Health Visitor and Midwife Should Know about the Children Act*, HMSO, Haywood, Manchester.

Shelley, P. (1991) A commitment to children. *Paediatric Nursing*, 3(7), 10–11.

Steele, B. (1980) Psychodynamic factors in child abuse, in *The Battered Child*, (eds C.H. Kempe and R.E. Helfer), University of Chicago Press, Chicago.

Thomas, D. (1991) How to deal with children in the emergency department. *Journal of Emergency Nursing*, 17(1), 49–50.

Toohey, S. and Field, P.A. (1985) Accident and Emergency. Parents' perceptions of care. *Nursing Mirror*, 161(19), 38–40.

Webb, J. and Cleaver, K. (1991) The child in casualty. *Nursing Times*, 87(5), 27–9.

Wordsworth, W. (1960) Intimations of Immortality, in *The Albatross Book of Verse*, 2nd edn, Collins, London, pp. 316–20.

Critical incident technique form

Ref/A&E/Critical Incident Technique no. ....

PLEASE NOTE: Information is collected via observation of an incident. Information should be collected by a person familiar with the action taking place, i.e. a colleague.

PART ONE: to be completed by the OBSERVER:

Name ....

Date ....

1 Describe the SITUATION observed.

....

....

2 The situation should now be broken down into a series of EVENTS/ ACTIVITIES. These should be described below and include the persons involved/associated with each event/activity.

....

....

3 Describe the area where the observed SITUATION took place.

....

4 For how long did you observe the situation?

....

....

5 Describe the outcome of the SITUATION.

....

....

6 Were observed actions effective/non-effective? Please give reasons.

....

....

7 Additional comments.

....

....

END OF PART ONE: Signature ....

                   Time ....

PART TWO: to be completed by all involved in the situation observed

Names ....

Date ....

Taking into consideration information recorded in Part One, identify the following:

1 What was the SITUATION observed?

....

....

2 Indicate any identified problems/issues associated with the SITUATION.

....

....

3 Identify the ACTION (by nurse/patient/others) that should have been taken within the observed SITUATION (this may be the same as that observed).

....

....

4 Break down the ACTION into smaller components/activities/events and identify which should have been undertaken by the nurse, by the patient, by others.

....

....

5 Convert information in 4 into a diagram (network) over the page.

6 Examine the network and indicate on the diagram the length of time required to complete each event.

7 Examine the network. Does this agree with Part Two, No. 4 YES/NO? If YES move on to Part Two, No. 9; if NO outline an approach to nursing action required to deal with the problem.

....

....

8 Discuss with colleagues and review the approach with reference to the network.

9 The action/s should now be evaluated in practice, information should be collected by a person familiar with the action taking place, i.e. a colleague.

10 Compare the new action with the network, discuss with colleagues similarities and differences and repeat the process accordingly commencing at stage 1, part 1.

11 Additional comments.

....

....

End of PART TWO

Signatures ....

....

Time ....

North Staffordshire Health Authority Adequate Care of the Elderly Guidelines

(Reprinted with the kind permission of North Staffordshire Health Authority)

GUIDELINES FOR STAFF

1. Recognition

It is important to recognize any change in the health and well-being of any elderly person and to document the facts carefully. In assessing the elderly person the possibility of inadequate care should be considered.

2. Report to manager

The information recorded should be reported and discussed with the manager who will make the decision to refer or not to refer.

3. Initial referral

3.1 The aim is for every referred incident of inadequate care of an elderly person of a serious nature to be treated with the same urgency as that accorded to incidents of child abuse by the duty officer of the relevant district or the hospital social work manager.

3.2 The following information should be obtained on receipt of a referral of suspected inadequate care of an elderly person:

3.2.1 The person's name, address, postcode, telephone number, age, gender and ethnic background (with language spoken if not from the indigenous population).

3.2.2 Description of alleged inadequate care, distinguishing clearly between what is suspected and what there is current evidence for. (Date of prior contacts, action taken and by whom are very helpful.)

3.2.3 General practitioner's name and telephone number and names and contact numbers for other relevant professionals involved.

3.2.4 The elderly person's close relatives and friends and their telephone numbers, relevant contacts from other agencies involved and their telephone numbers.

3.2.5 Alleged abuser's name, address and telephone number, physical description and knowledge of his/her behaviour, relationship to elderly person and length of relationship.

3.2.6 Referrer's name and contact telephone number, description of referrer's involvement in case to date and how long referrer has known elderly person (referrers may in some circumstances wish to remain anonymous, but referrals will nonetheless be investigated). All referrers giving their name should be warned at the time of referral that their evidence may be needed if they have reported a crime.

3.3 In both an emergency and where there is reasonable cause to suspect inadequate care, staff should focus their concern on the elderly person and initiate action.

4. Investigation

The professional involved should:

4.1 check with other agencies as to whether the elderly person or alleged abuser is known and under what circumstances;

4.2 visit accompanied by another worker if circumstances indicate that such precautions are appropriate;

4.3 interview the dependent elderly person alone without the caregiver and in circumstances in which the elderly person is certain of privacy;

4.4 explain to the caregiver that he/she will be interviewed separately after the elderly person has been interviewed and that this is normal departmental practice;

4.5 make a preliminary assessment of the mental capacity of the dependent elderly person;

4.6   pay special attention to suspicious signs and symptoms and precipitating factors;

4.7   work assessment questions into conversation in a relaxed manner and do not rush the elderly person or the caregiver during the interview (if the interpreting services are required, care must be taken to ensure that the interpreter is someone independent of the elderly person's family and recognized as competent to fulfil this role);

4.8   keep accurate factual notes on any injuries observed, who was present at the interview, what was said, what explanations were given, the group dynamics, and any other relevant events. These are necessary to help in management;

4.9   where appropriate, carry out a full assessment including nutritional status, and emotional status, in addition to the full documentation of injuries.

5. Subsequent action

5.1   Referral should be made to the client's general practitioner or appropriate hospital medical staff so that a medical examination of the elderly person can be made immediately, with the informed consent of the elderly person. If injuries are found they should be mapped on a body chart.

5.2   Arrangements to protect an elderly person at risk must be made as soon as possible. A multidisciplinary case conference (involving wherever possible the elderly person and caregiver) should be arranged within 72 hours and held within ten days. At this conference information will be fully shared, action planned and a careful record made of the investigation and subsequent action taken.
       A key worker may be identified and thereafter all staff should communicate relevant information and anxieties to the key worker.
       The confidential nature of all reports should be respected.

5.3   If there is urgent need to protect an inadequately cared for elderly person such an elderly person will have priority for allocation of a place in a residential unit, provided he/she is willing to be admitted. If medical care or an opinion as to the elderly person's competence to make such a decision is required, negotiations should be urgently undertaken through the elderly person's GP, or appropriate hospital medical staff, to obtain this.

5.4   In appropriate cases the police should be informed if it is suspected that a crime has been committed against person or property.

6. Records

Due attention must be paid to maintaining a high standard of documentation.

7. Remember

Many cases will present:

- as suspicion rather than 'proof';
- not as an emergency or a dramatic event, but as an insidious development.

Most cases will require ongoing and patient casework with the objective of improving the adequacy of care.

INFORMATION FOR STAFF

Attitudes of society to the elderly

Major social changes are occurring which have a profound effect on the lives of all, both young and old.

It is important to examine the attitudes of society towards the older generation, their role in society and the provision of the help required if so determined.

The term 'granny battering' is emotive and incorrect in that it is based on an ageist and sexist view of elderly people. This view perceives the old as dear little whitehaired grannies whose only role in life is to placidly dote on their adoring grandchildren.

The belief that families do not care for elderly people is a variant on the more general belief that there was an era before the Industrial Revolution in which elderly people were loved, respected and cared for by relatives and neighbours. This belief is a myth and the belief that families cared better in the past is also untrue.

An accompaniment to the ageing process is a loss of power and status and deprivation in terms of both income and other resources.

The physical abuse of frail and/or elderly people is not new although many find it hard to believe that carers/relatives are capable of inflicting harm. Furthermore, it is sometimes extremely difficult to recognize a person who is being injured and minor injuries can be a prelude to more severe injuries.

It could be considered that some cases of neglect can be thought of as inadequate care defined as the presence of unmet needs for personal care. These needs include all basic requirements as well as those of supportive relationships, the opportunity to define an acceptable lifestyle and freedom from all forms of violence.

Most definitions of inadequate care include the following eight categories.

1. *Assault*

Repeated occurrences of 'falls' or injuries that cannot be explained adequately and to the satisfaction of the doctor should be viewed with suspicion.

Injuries which should receive special attention are:

- bruises to face and arms;
- welts;
- lacerations;
- fractures;
- burns;
- signs of hair pulling, e.g. haemorrhage below the scalp.

2. *Deprivation of nutrition*

Unless severe this may be difficult to identify, particularly as the older person may forget when he/she last ate and make false allegations of starvation. One useful indicator is where the carer is also neglecting him/herself by not eating.

Signs may include:

- dry skin;
- sunken eyes;
- weight loss.

3. *Administration of inappropriate drugs or deprivation of prescribed drugs*

The older person may be given an extra sleeping tablet in order that the carer will get a good night's sleep. However, this can progress to the elderly person regularly receiving double or treble the prescribed dose. Situations can arise in which additional medication is used as an inappropriate control measure:

Possible indicators include:

- excessive drowsiness;
- apathy;
- incontinence;
- dehydration.

4. *Emotional*

Inflicting mental anguish on an older person includes the use of threatening remarks, insults, harsh comments, isolation from social contact, treating the older person as being invisible and consistently ignoring his/her concerns or comments.

Possible indicators include:

- insomnia, sleep deprivation or need for excessive sleep;
- change in appetite;
- unusual weight gain or loss;
- tearfulness;
- unexplained paranoia;
- low self-esteem;
- excessive fears;
- ambivalence;
- confusion;
- resignation;
- agitation.

5. Sexual abuse

Any form of sexual contact or exposure without the older person's consent or when the older person is incapable of giving adequate consent is abuse.

Possible signs or symptoms include:

- stained or bloody underclothing;
- pain in the genital area;
- bruises or bleeding in external genitalia, vaginal or anal areas;
- sexually transmitted diseases.

6. Deprivation of help in performing activities of daily living

This can be mistaken for self-neglect particularly when the carer does not live in the same house as the older person.

Signs which should alert the professional include:

- hypothermia/hyperthermia;
- absence of glasses, hearing aid, dentures or prosthesis;
- unexpected or unexplained deterioration of health;
- pressure sores.

7. Involuntary isolation and confinement

This may be initiated as a safety measure but becomes inappropriate control, e.g. to prevent the older person falling out of his/her chair a carer may tie him/her to the chair or jam a table up to the chair. This control may result in injuries such as rope burns or bruising to the legs or shins.

Doors may be locked and the resulting isolation may include the rejection of contact with outside agencies.

8. Financial abuse

This type of abuse includes the misuse or exploitation of or inattention to an older person's possessions and/or funds. Forms of this include conning or threatening the older person into handing over assets, abusing or neglecting the responsibility to manage the older person's money and stealing possessions or cash.

Possible indicators include:

- unexplained or sudden inability to pay bills;
- unexplained or sudden withdrawal of money from accounts;
- disparity between assets and satisfactory living conditions;
- lack of receptivity by older person, or carer, to any necessary assistance requiring expenditure when finances are not a problem;
- extraordinary interest by family members in an older person's assets.

Factors associated with increased risk

Research has identified some major factors which, when present, can assist workers in identifying elderly people who are at increased risk of mistreatment. Staff should therefore consider the following:

1. Psychosocial history

Do any of the children or other relatives in contact with the elderly person have a history of mental illness? Is there a tendency towards acting out aggression? Are there signs of alcohol and/or drug misuse?

2. Transgenerational violence

Is there a past history of violence in the family?

3. Dependency

Is there an adult, child or other person in the home dependent on the older person for income, shelter or emotional support?

4. Stress

Have any stressful life events occurred recently, for example, loss of job, moving, death of a significant other? Is there chronic financial stress? Is there an opportunity of respite for the carers?

5. *Isolation*

Does the older person have a satisfactory amount and quality of contact with family, friends and neighbours? Does the older person have the opportunity to pursue interests outside the home?

6. *Living arrangements*

Does the older person share his or her home with other people or does the older person live with a family in their home?

Inadequate care

Definitions are a great problem. Eastman uses the word 'abuse' and speaks of emotional and psychological abuse of an older person by a formal or informal carer. The abuse is repeated and is the violation of a person's human and civil rights by a person or persons who have power over the life of a dependent.

Elder abuse has also been defined as 'the actions of a caretaker which create unmet needs for the elderly person'. Neglect can be defined as 'the failure of an individual responsible for caretaking to respond adequately to established needs for care'.

Research and experience have shown that the use of the phrase 'inadequate care' has resulted in significant advantages, in that it is easier to agree on what is adequate or inadequate care than what is acceptable or unacceptable behaviour. There is much less reluctance to identify inadequate care than to categorize the problem as abuse or neglect.

The victim

The focus of attention has been on the characteristics of the 'victim' who is typically:

- elderly (over age 75);
- female;
- roleless;
- functionally impaired;
- lonely;
- fearful;
- living at home with an adult child.

and often:

- heavy;
- immobile;
- incontinent;
- has negative personality traits.

The abusers

Recent research has, however, concentrated on the abusers who tended to be sons. Psychological abuse predominated and was followed in frequency by physical abuse. These abusers were likely to be dependent on the victim for finances, led stressful lives and had health and financial problems. One-third had psychological difficulties and even more had a history of mental illness and alcohol abuse. Professional intervention should therefore be activated in these situations.

All carers may be in need of vital help and this should be actioned by referral to voluntary agencies/statutory services.

The abuse will continue as long as the abuser gains from it. When the 'exchange' becomes unfavourable, e.g. through guilt, professional intervention, etc., the abuse ceases.

Associated factors

Some factors associated with increased risk of inadequate care may include:

- poor communication or breakdown of communication;
- perception of carer of the dependence of the older person;
- frequent visits to general practitioners by the informal carers to talk about their problems;
- role reversal;
- history of falls and minor injuries;
- triggering behaviour – an incident that acts as a catalyst inducing loss of control;
- carer's and dependent's apathy;
- cramped or substandard living conditions;
- those with chronic progressive, disabling illnesses that impair function and create care needs and exceed or will exceed their carer's ability to meet them, such as:
  - dementia
  - Parkinsonism
  - severe arthritis
  - severe cardiac disease
  - severe chronic lung disease
  - severe diabetes mellitus
  - recurrent strokes;
- those with progressive impairments who are without informal support from family or neighbours or whose caretakers manifest signs of 'burn-out';
- those residing in institutions that have a history of providing substandard care;

- those whose caretakers are under sudden increased stress due, for example, to loss of job, health or spouse.

Recognition

This can be very difficult because some ageing processes can cause changes which are hard to distinguish from some aspects of physical assault, e.g. skin bruising can occur very easily due to blood vessels becoming very fragile.

The presence of one or more of the features of inadequate care identified earlier does not establish the case, they merely alert one to the possibility.

Preventative measures

1. Caring for the carers

Caring for the elderly at home involves a great deal of stress and has little support or recognition. It can take over the whole of the individual's life and they can become invisible and isolated with financial, physical and emotional problems.

They require help in four dimensions:

1. Practical. Help with household and personal care tasks and finances.
2. Behavioural. Assistance to respond to incontinence, unsafe acts, wandering, disturbance of sleep at night.
3. Interpersonal. Support in dealing with sadness at changes in the relative, loss of tolerance and tension in the household.
4. Social. Measures to limit restrictions on getting out, seeing family and friends, holidays and going out to work.

Without adequate help these stresses can build up and lead to inadequate care of the elderly person although the carers can in fact be abused themselves.

2. Carer's Charter

There is a Carer's Charter available from Age Concern which spells out ten points:

1. *Recognition* – of their contribution and of their own needs as individuals in their own right.
2. *Services* – tailored to their individual circumstances, needs and views, through discussion at the time help is being planned.

3. *Services* – which reflect an awareness of differing racial, cultural and religious backgrounds and values, equally accessible to carers of every race and ethnic origin.
4. *Opportunities* – for a break, both for short spells (an afternoon) and for longer periods (a week or more), to relax and have time to themselves.
5. *Practical* – help to lighten the tasks of caring, including domestic help, home adaptation, incontinence services and help with transport.
6. *Someone* – to talk to about their own emotional needs, at the outset of caring, while they are caring and when the caring task is over.
7. *Information* – about available benefits and services as well as how to cope with the particular conditions of the person cared for.
8. *An income* – which covers the costs of caring and which does not preclude carers' taking employment or sharing care with other people.
9. *Opportunities* – to explore alternatives to family care, both for the immediate and long term future.
10. *Services* – designed through consultation with carers at all levels of policy planning.

3. Advocacy

The forms of advocacy are:

- legal advocacy;
- self-advocacy;
- group advocacy.

Citizen's advocacy exists to help frail and vulnerable elderly people in a number of ways. It is when an individual enters into a relationship with an elderly person and represents the interest of that person who needs help and assistance to improve their quality of life and have the appropriate entitlements. The advocate provides emotional support through friendship and enables the individual to have benefits of all kinds. The advocate can assist in preventing inadequate care.

Intervention

In extreme cases it may be necessary to invoke legal proceedings. The need to do this should always be discussed in detail with a senior manager.

Inadequate care in an institutional setting

There are two different aspects of this:

1. There is abuse of the individual, e.g. when the person is hit, verbally abused or has their money stolen or misused.
2. There is inadequate care that arises from elderly people being subject to regimes which deny their individuality and deprive them of the quality of life.

It is essential to have Codes of Practice for residential care and to have the patients and relatives at the centre of activity, with well-developed individual care programmes meeting the specified and assessed needs of individuals. The monitoring of the quality of care will be based on that agreed plan. There must also be an emphasis on the ongoing education and training of staff.

Education and training

Education and training are required to allow staff to fully understand and discuss the issue of adequate care of elderly people. Managers need to be trained to recognize their responsibility to staff to support them in handling the complex situations that can develop in the identification of inadequate care and responding to it.

Elderly care nursing assessment form

Presenting problem:

Pre-existing conditions:

Medication:

Accommodation:
Patient lives alone
With spouse
With family
Lives in warden controlled accommodation
Residential/nursing home

Support available:

Dependency:

Self-caring

Requires help to:
Bath
Wash
Dress
Feed
Toilet

Mobility:
Fully mobile
Requires help to walk and stand
Bed fast

Mobility aids:
Walking stick
Zimmer frame
Tripod

Sensory Status

Vision:
Good
Uses spectacles
Blind

Hearing:
Hearing aid
Deaf

Mental State:
Alert
Confused at times
Confused
Disorientated
Aggressive

Lifestyle:
Smokes
Drinks

Discharge from Accident and Emergency

Date Admitted:

Discharge home, no extra support required:

Discharge home, referrals made to:
GP
HV
DN
CPN
Meals on Wheels
Social Services
Age Concern
Other agencies (name)

Additional comments:

Signature:

Index